THE LIVE LONGER NOW

Quick Weight-Loss Program

THE
LIVE LONGER
NOW
Quick
Weight-Loss
Program

by Jon N. Leonard, Ph.D.

GROSSET & DUNLAP
A FILMWAYS COMPANY
Publishers • New York

The author and publishers wish to remind you
that it is sound practice to consult your doctor
before beginning any new dietary program.

I dedicate this book to my parents, whose wisdom has guided me and whose love has supported me through my life.

Acknowledgments

Human obesity is a field of research that is finally receiving the attention it deserves. In recent years great strides have been made in our understanding of obesity. Philip Balch, Albert Stunkard, Jean Mayer, S. Schacter, Richard Stuart, and others too numerous to mention have contributed important pieces to the puzzle. Their contributions have formed a basis without which this book could not have been written. I acknowledge with humility the great debt I owe these outstanding researchers. To the extent this book achieves its lofty goal, which is to reduce the incidence of obesity in modern society, these people deserve much of the credit. To the extent that it does not achieve this goal, since it is a creation of mine alone, I am fully responsible.

I also wish to acknowledge the many people who have been directly or indirectly involved in the writing of this book: my wife Nadine Leonard, Marie Di Meglio, Peggy Hunter, Marty Helin, Lucinda Sanchez, Ralph Stevenson, my children, the guests of the Institute of Health, and many others. To them all, my sincere thanks.

Contents

Introduction

A laboratory rat is a marvelous creature that lives its life in the scientist's controlled environment. What happens when we remove the rat from the laboratory, take it home, make a pet of it, and feed it plenty of what it likes to eat? The rat becomes obese.

In the labs of the Psychology Department of Brooklyn College, Sclafani and Springer showed that rats enjoy eating just as much as humans do. In a landmark experiment, normal adult rats were given free access to a variety of highly palatable supermarket foods like salami, cookies, cheese, and peanut butter, as well as their normal feed. The rats chose to eat predominantly supermarket foods, and they ate voraciously. Within two months they were more than 50 percent overweight.

Like Sclafani and Springer's rats, we have access to an almost limitless supply of highly palatable supermarket foods. And as with the rats, our indulgence in these foods produces obesity in us. It has been estimated that as many as 80 million Americans are obese, and in spite of a national interest in weight loss the problem of obesity continues to grow as the list of highly palatable foods at the supermarket seems to grow year by year.

Actually the idea that "highly palatable" foods cause overweight is somewhat misleading. Few would deny that fresh cucumbers, lettuce, tomatoes, and other delicious foods are highly palatable. Yet these are not foods that lead to overweight.

The problem is that "palatable" simply means delicious, and it is not deliciousness per se that leads to overeating. Some delicious foods, such as calorically dilute vegetables, do not lend themselves to overeating. Even some foods that are more calorically intense, such as whole grains, do not readily lend themselves to overeating.

So rather than use an old word that doesn't work well, I prefer to use the new variation, "palatation," in the descriptive phrase "high palatation level," to describe foods like salami, cookies, cheese, and peanut butter, which readily lend themselves to overeating. Thus these foods would be said to have a high palatation level. On the other hand, delicious foods like cucumbers, lettuce, and tomatoes, which do not readily lend themselves to overeating, would be said to have a low palatation level. This convention will be used throughout the book, and its utility will become apparent.

By definition, then, high palatation foods are those foods that lend themselves to overeating and overweight. Because such foods combine several characteristics, including deliciousness, caloric intensity, and perhaps rapid absorption in the gut, this definition of high palatation implicitly carries the same characteristics.

This definition, which is intended to be used intuitively, makes an important distinction among foods. The best examples of high palatation foods I know of are blends of sugars and fats in the marvelous desserts that abound in our eating environment. The palatation level of these foods is so high that even lean individuals can be induced to eat tremendous quantities of them. Sims and his collaborators from the University of Vermont and elsewhere showed that men of normal weight could be induced to eat in excess of 10,000 calories per day indefinitely. Substantial experimental obesity could be produced in this manner.

Sims' data also showed that dietary fat independently worsened the sugar tolerances of these subjects. In addition, it produced high levels of blood insulin in them. The fact that high fat worsens sugar tolerance and elevates blood insulin has been known since the classical work of Himsworth with nondiabetics and diabetics nearly fifty years ago.

Sugars, or more precisely, simple carbohydrates, have been shown by numerous investigators to produce exaggerated insulin and blood sugar responses when compared with complex carbohydrates such as fruits, vegetables, and other foods as grown. A recent report in the *Lancet* disclosed that even apple juice produces exaggerated insulin and sugar responses when compared with the intact apple, due to the liberation of fruit sugar by the juicing process.

Thus high palatation foods, sugar and fat, produce abnormal sugar tolerances and elevated insulin levels in people of normal weight.

And a common characteristic of the overweight person is an abnormal sugar tolerance and an elevated blood insulin level. In other words, high palatation levels produce in normal people the same blood disturbances seen in obese people. This may not be coincidental.

The eating behavior of overweight people is alarmingly suggestive of a disturbance in the brain's hypothalamic satiety center. While hypothalamic tumor or other specific damage to the hypothalamus causes obesity only in rare instances, the likelihood is high that a poorly functioning satiety center is part and parcel of obesity. The satiety center's nerve cells are known to be stimulated by both the insulin level in the blood and the rate of sugar uptake in the body. The abnormal insulin levels and abnormal sugar uptakes associated with high palatation foods may well affect the satiety center's ability to respond adequately to control the intake of foods on a day-to-day basis. Such a direct effect of high palatation foods on the satiety center would certainly help account for the incredible prevalence of obesity in our culture. And the obese individual's chronically abnormal insulin and sugar uptake would act to perpetuate the satiety center's disability and increase the likelihood of his or her remaining obese.

The brain's satiety center is crucial in controlling food intake. Overeating and obesity are the direct outcomes of damage to this center.

Damage to the satiety center produces remarkable and distinctive behavior. In 1950 Neal Miller first reported the eating behavior of rats whose satiety centers had been destroyed. Of course, they overate and became fat. Beyond that, the cardinal feature of these rats was that *impediments* to eating caused a reduction in the amount they ate. The rats would eat if food was freely available, but if they had to work for it by pressing a bar or lifting a cover, or if eating was made unpleasant, the rats would greatly reduce their food intake. This finicky behavior proved characteristic of all obese rats whose obesity was the result of satiety center disablement.

Sclafani and Springer showed that the same finicky behavior is exhibited by rats who become obese solely by overeating high palatation supermarket foods. Their satiety centers had not been damaged, and yet the behavior prevailed. It is hard to imagine that this distinctive behavior can result from any cause other than a reduced level of functioning of the satiety center.

Obese humans exhibit a behavior analogous to that of the rat whose satiety center has been impaired. While testing humans on a complex behavior like eating presents great difficulties, numerous ingenious studies have been done. Schacter and his associates, for example, observed nearly 500 customers of 14 Oriental restaurants to determine whether the obese customers were more or less likely to go to the trouble of using chopsticks than the nonobese. (Ninety percent of the customers were Westerners and presumably unaccustomed to the use of chopsticks.) Schacter found that obese customers were far less likely to take the trouble to use chopsticks than were persons of normal weight. In another study, this one at St. Luke's Hospital in New York City, Hashim and Van Itallie showed that an obese individual is far less likely to consume an adequate amount of calories when given a relatively bland formula diet than is a person of normal weight. Many other studies have demonstrated eating behaviors in obese humans analogous to the finicky eating habits of the obese rat.

It is tempting to believe that the obese human's finicky eating behavior is related to a degraded function of the hypothalamic satiety center. Blood disturbances that would tend to adversely affect the proper functioning of the satiety center are present in the obese person, as we mentioned. And the fact that these same blood disturbances are produced by high palatation foods, sugars and fats abundantly available in our modern diet, might help explain the prevalence of obesity in modern society.

Not all cultures have a degree of obesity as high as that found in modern Western cultures. Epidemiological studies have shown that native cultures around the world generally have an absence of obesity. The Bantus of Africa, who until very recently were relatively untouched by modern culture, enjoy an astonishingly low incidence of obesity. The native diet is the paradigm of low palatation food: cereals, grains, and vegetables; less than 10 percent of total calories comes from fat, and little from sugar. The 50,000 Tarahumara Indians of northern Mexico are a recently studied native population that has excited great interest because of their continued isolation from civilization. Connor and his associates reported a virtual absence of obesity among these Indians, as well as an absence of degenerative diseases such as heart disease and high blood pressure. Again, the Tarahumara diet is of the low palatation variety: beans, corn, vegetables, little animal products, and a total fat intake of about 12 percent.

A Bantu or Tarahumara native must consume 4.5 pounds of food in order to get his 2000 calories each day. The Western individual, eating "modern" food, needs to consume only 1.9 pounds in order to get the same 2000 calories. Thus Western foods, bite for bite, are 232 percent as calorically intense as the foods of these native cultures. This high caloric intensity is a key factor in the high palatation level of Western foods and is not a factor in the food of native cultures.

Without question, obesity depends on food habits. And because food habits are culturally related, obesity also strongly depends on culture.

In 1962 Srole and collaborators reported their findings after a systematic study of 110,000 people in New York City. They found that obesity in this population, especially among women, was strongly related to socioeconomic status: the lower the socioeconomic status, the greater the prevalence of obesity. Dividing socioeconomic status into high, medium, and low, they found that obesity in the low-status group was six times as prevalent as obesity in the high-status group. Fully 30 percent of the low-status women were obese, whereas no more than 5 percent of the high-status women exceeded normal weight limits. The middle-status group fell in between; about 16 percent were overweight.

Does low income create obesity? Not at all. A study of American Navajo children by Stunkard and Garb compared obesity rates in children reared in modern Western ways (acculturated) with those reared traditionally (unacculturated). Obesity in the acculturated child was much higher than in the unacculturated child, reflecting the different food habits of the ancient Navajo culture from those of the modern culture many Navajos have adopted. Since the unacculturated Navajo lives at a substantially lower income level than the acculturated Navajo, we have an example of less obesity at less income—just the opposite of the New York findings.

Oscanova, who is at the Institute of Epidemiology in Prague, Czechoslovakia, reports a change in obesity that occurred in Czechoslovakia in the fifteen years from 1956 to 1971. By 1971 the prevalence of obesity (defined as 125 percent of ideal weight) had increased 20 percent for men and 30 percent for women. Over the same fifteen years, the average caloric intake of an individual had increased 20 percent and the fat intake (mostly from animal products) had increased 50 percent. Also, leisure time increased and physical activity decreased among the general population.

It may be easiest to see the strong effect that culture has on obesity by examining some cultural beliefs different from our own. In Nigeria, fats and oils are discouraged in the diet of women until after thay have borne a child and are lactating. Then women are encouraged to eat fats and oils in the belief that lactation will be improved. As a result of this practice, there is a surge in the incidence of obesity in women between the ages of 25 and 35, when lactation is most frequent, and a trailing off of obesity before and after those ages.

An example of bizarre food habits occurs among Japanese Sumo wrestlers. In a sport where body size carries a tremendous advantage, the prevalence of obesity is nearly 100 percent. Caloric intake ranges between 5000 and 6000 calories per day of foods of the highest palatation levels. Kuzuya and his collaborators reported that nearly half of the 550 wrestlers surveyed had weight indices between 30 and 70 percent above normal. Some were as much as 100 percent over normal weight. Kuzuya also showed that the Sumo wrestler's obesity predisposed him to degenerative disease: 60 percent of the active wrestlers over 20 years old had diabetic glucose tolerance tests.

We don't think of our own food habits as bizarre. Yet in an important way they are. The U.S. Department of Agriculture has put out a 190-page handbook called *Composition of Foods* that shows the nutrient composition of thousands of common foods. This handbook is absolutely amazing, not because it shows the nutrients in foods, but because it lists what it considers "common" foods. This list is replete with pies, meat cuts, pastries, cakes, and other high palatation preparations. The fundamental entries for vegetables, grains, fruits and other *basic* foods form a very small part of this huge list of foods. If a Tarahumaran were to look at this list, he would find it very strange. And I think it would be immediately apparent to him that the obesity in our culture is related to the bizarre food habits we have.

Although this book is not about diabetes, high blood pressure, heart attacks, or any other degenerative diseases, it is worth noting that these conditions, like obesity, are cultural phenomena strongly related to diet. The overconsumption of fat, sugar, salt, and cholesterol has been related to five of the top killer diseases in the United States: heart disease, cancer, stroke, atherosclerosis, and diabetes. In testimony before the U.S. Senate, Dr. Mark Hegsted of the Harvard School of Public Health said:

> I wish to stress that there is a great deal of evidence and it continues to accumulate, which strongly implicates and, in some instances, proves that the major causes of death and disability in the United States are related to the diet we eat. I include coronary artery disease which accounts for nearly half of the deaths in the United States, several of the most important forms of cancer, hypertension, diabetes and obesity as well as other chronic diseases.

After hearing testimony from hundreds of the world's top nutrition and health specialists and reviewing thousands of pages of documentation, the Senate's Select Committee on Nutrition published the first set of dietary goals ever promulgated by a federal agency for the United States as a whole. These goals strive to reduce fat consumption (all fats, including unsaturated fats) by 30 percent, to cut sugar consumption drastically, and to increase complex carbohydrate consumption so as to make it the greatest portion of the daily food intake. These goals would shift American eating habits in the direction of those of the Tarahumara, the Bantu, and other groups whose incidences of obesity and degenerative diseases are rare to nonexistent.

The Institute of Health in Tucson, Arizona, is one of the few institutions in the United States that uses a diet similar to these native cultures as part of its treatment of obesity and degenerative disease. As the institute's director, I have had an opportunity to see firsthand the dramatic effect such a radical change in diet can have. The influencible risk factors associated with diabetes, high blood pressure, and heart disease can be rapidly and drastically altered with such a diet. Cholesterol level, blood pressure level, and blood triglyceride levels usually fall to normal levels in 20 to 60 days. The low palatation level inherent in this diet greatly increases the ease with which the risk factor "obesity" can be treated. A steady-state weight loss of a pound a week can be maintained without discomfort.

I would be the last to say that we know all that needs to be known about obesity and the complex human behavior called eating that induces it. Yet we do know enough to cure the condition. We know that obesity is directly related to the food we eat. We know that when we allow ourselves (or our pet mouse) free access to the high palatation foods of modern culture, obesity becomes a threat (to both man and mouse). And we know that if we were to limit ourselves to the low or medium palatation foods of many native cultures, obesity would disappear.

As humans, we are free to choose the foods we eat, allowing what we may and restricting what we decide to restrict. At the Institute of Health, we have found that informed people are willing to make the personal choice of an eating style that offers improved health and a more suitable body weight.

The way I see it, there really isn't any choice if we wish to avoid degenerative disease and early death. An improved diet is the only practical way to avoid these diseases. Achieving an optimal body weight may be viewed as merely a bonus.

The focus of this book is on teaching an eating style for the control of overweight. Nevertheless, two other aspects of overweight cannot be overlooked. One is the lack of physical activity, which contributes to overweight. And the other is the eating situation around us, which needs to be managed if we are to be successful in weight loss. Therefore, physical activity and situational management are a part of the overall program taught in this book.

CHAPTER 1

Read This Chapter First

This book is a result of my work at the Institute of Health, a health service organization in Tucson, Arizona, on a new food program that is proving to be a major advance in the control of overweight. The diet described in this book was designed in the early 1970s by the Longevity Foundation of America in San Pedro, California. It is derived from the diet of native cultures but is suitable for use by modern man. It is patterned after the Bantu/Tarahumara diet: plenty of complex carbohydrates (vegetables, fruits, and grains) and very low levels of fat, sugar, salt, and cholesterol. It is a high-fiber diet emphasizing foods as grown and deemphasizing foods that have been substantially processed. It is an inexpensive diet with a high nutrient level.

The food program and a cooking technology to go with it have been described in the two books *Live Longer Now* and *The Live Longer Now Cookbook*. The program is called the Live Longer Now Diet Program, or the longevity food program.

In this book I am interested in the Live Longer Now diet only as a tool for weight loss, *the quickest possible weight loss* compatible with long-term success. The diet is integrated with physical activity and situational management in an overall program that I call the Live Longer Now Quick Weight-Loss Program.

There's a Problem Here Someplace

Of the 80 million Americans who are obese, two-thirds are dieting to lose weight. Very few of these dieters will be successful. Even under controlled clinical conditions the situation is dismal. Witness these conclusions of the Cornell Conferences on Therapy:

> . . . most obese patients will not remain in treatment. Of those who do, most will not lose significant poundage, and of those who do lose weight, most will regain it promptly.

With all the weight-loss books, clinics, and programs in existence today you would think obesity would be a declining problem in our society. It is not. If anything, it is increasing.

Why do weight-loss programs have such poor success rates? Why does lost weight return? Why are many weight-loss programs successful only at the expense of general health?

All these questions have a common answer: In our society, the foods we have at our disposal predispose to obesity, and the foods that would prevent obesity are not widely consumed or available. Native population groups, on the other hand, whose cultural habits lead them to eat foods that fall within the sphere of "longevity foods," can maintain perfect body weight without the benefit of weight-loss programs of any kind.

We all know the many reducing techniques used in America. Do any of them work? Look outside your window at the overfat people walking by and you will have your answer. Americans are so interested in reducing unwanted fat, that if any one of the hundreds of reducing techniques were truly effective, fatness would virtually disappear.

Now, in your mind take a trip to the Sierra Madre of northern Mexico and take a look at the Tarahumara Indians living there. Their weight-control technique is simply to follow the eating habits of their ancient culture. Does it work? Yes. Obesity is virtually absent among the Tarahumaras. If you investigated the Bantu natives of southern Africa you would see similar eating habits and the same result: no obesity. In these native diets, you have a reducing program that really works—and a prescription for your own eating habits.

If you are willing to change the way you eat—permanently—you can become and stay slim. The process is simple and painless. You won't go hungry and you won't deprive yourself of food. In fact, you will be eating a supernutritious diet. You will have to adjust your taste buds, you will have to do a little work, and you will have to do some thinking. This book will show you, step by step, how to go about it.

If you're not willing to make a permanent change in the way you eat, then I'm afraid you will have to remain fat. Or what is worse for your health, you will join the roller-coaster plan of weight control: up and down the scales as you move from one diet to another, constantly striving, never succeeding, living your life in a permanent program of failure.

You may feel picked on because you are overweight and have to change the way you eat, while people who aren't overweight can eat anything they please. The truth is, people of normal weight need the Live Longer Now program just as much as you do. Their health and their lives are critically affected by the foods they eat. By not making a dietary change, they are unknowingly sentencing themselves to a shorter, sicker life than they could have had.

You might consider yourself lucky. You have a visible symptom, your overweight, that has prompted you to undertake the Live Longer Now program. Without this symptom, normal-weight people may never be stimulated to make a move that would lead to a longer, healthier life. Yet, if they had any sense, they would do exactly what you are setting out to do.

Some Top Nutritionists Are Wrong

Some nutritionists maintain that there is nothing wrong with the American diet. They say it is not only excellent but perhaps the best diet humans have ever had. I do not agree. And I think the obvious evidence argues against it.

Eighty million obese Americans, a million deaths a year from heart and related diseases, and an adult life expectancy in America less than that in primitive cultures* all argue against these claims for our diet. Fortunately, most people don't subscribe to these claims either.

In the past few years we have had a chance to see what benefits can come from even modest changes in a nation's diet. Since the publica-

---

*The average 40-year-old American has less likelihood of reaching 50 than the average 40-year-old in most developing nations.

tion of the first Live Longer Now book, and as a result of the interest of many groups in modifying American diets by reducing sugar, fat, and salt and increasing the amount of vegetable and grain intake, some significant things have happened. For the first time since records have been kept, heart disease has actually declined slightly; and for the first time since the 1940s, the life span has increased slightly in America.

The Palatation Level of Foods

The term palatation level is used frequently in this book. By palatation level of a food, I mean the extent to which a food leads to overeating and overweight. Chocolate chip cookies, for example, can be said to have a high palatation level for most people. In our culture high palatation foods abound; pies, cakes, french fries, choice-cut steaks, mayonnaise, butter, and oils would be on most people's lists.

Lettuce is a low palatation food for everyone. No one can overeat lettuce to the point of overweight. Many other vegetables are in the same category. Bean sprouts, beet greens, green beans, radishes, zucchine squash, and spinach are familiar examples. Foods that have a surprisingly low palatation level, given their high caloric density, are foods such as whole grains, beans, and corn. Fish, poultry, and lean meats also have *relatively* low palatation levels.

High palatation foods are the trademark of the modern Western culture, a culture in which obesity abounds. Low to medium palatation foods are the trademark of nonobese cultures, and these foods form the backbone of longevity eating.

Necessary and sufficient conditions for a food to be a high palatation food, and therefore conducive to overeating, are the following:

1. The food is calorically intense.
2. The food is capable of rapid absorption by the gut.
3. The food is delicious.

If any condition is absent, the food is not a likely candidate for overeating and therefore not a high palatation food. Any food that satisfies all three conditions surely is.

You might think that any delicious food that is calorically intense would be a high palatation food. But this does not seem to be the case. In order to qualify as a high palatation food, it must also be rapidly absorbable, as sugars and fats are.

Beans and whole grains are calorically intense foods that many people (I am one of them) find delicious. Yet if they are prepared simply and not milled, processed, or overcooked so as to render them "predigested" (and therefore too rapidly absorbed), they are not easily overeaten. That this is true is attested to by the fact that neither the patients at the Institute of Health, nor the Tarahumaras, nor anyone else who has adopted this style of eating will overeat these foods.

Consider this scenario: At the Institute of Health the evening meal, an excellent longevity lasagna, is over and everyone is sitting around the dining table. Marie is about to clear the table. But first she checks to see if anyone wants more. More lasagna, anyone? No thanks, Marie. How about more corn or vegetables? No thanks. More salad or bread? No thanks. It was delicious, but we are full. We are full and we know it. We are finished eating.

But are there foods that would induce us to eat even when we are full? Is that possible? You bet it is. And those foods are the high palatation ones: those delicious high caloric foods that are absorbed rapidly by the gut into the bloodstream.

See if this sounds familiar: Hungry? No, I'm full. Want a cookie? Umm . . . yeah, thanks.

The sugar in that cookie will be absorbed into your bloodstream within minutes. Sugar is predigested carbohydrate; it requires no digestion on your part. It will be absorbed partially through the roof of your mouth while you are still chewing and partially through your esophagus while you are still swallowing; then it will be rapidly finished off in your digestive tract.

Your body knows that it is getting a caloric bonanza from that cookie. It knows, from having been fed many cookies in the past, that within seconds a large quantity of calories will be captured, absorbed, and ready to be stored away (as fat) for a rainy day. Because "capturing calories" was an important survival trait in evolutionary man, the cookie is looked on by the body as a prize.

Your body's response to the offer of a cookie is to accept it (Umm . . . yeah, thanks) because it can use it with so little effort.

But more corn and beans on a full stomach? No, thanks. There's a lot of work to digesting and absorbing corn and beans, and there is plenty of digestion already going on.

Of course, if you add sugar or butter to the corn and beans, it's a different story. You've made at least some of each bite a rapidly absorbed food, and you just might accept the offer of more. Even salt, which acts like sugar in being highly prized by the body in spite of its overabundance in our food, can render another helping more acceptable to a full stomach.

Rapidly absorbed foods, especially sugars and fats, create an abnormal situation in the blood. Blood insulin and blood glucose behave abnormally in someone who consumes either a high sugar diet or a high fat diet. This is a cause for concern when it comes to overweight because the brain's hunger center (and therefore one's eating behavior) is controlled by the action of blood insulin and blood sugar. A disturbance in the hunger center can lead to obesity. And there is reason to believe that the blood glucose and insulin disturbances created by high palatation foods contribute directly to overeating (see page 2).

The Live Longer Now Diet

The Live Longer Now diet is characterized by

1. plenty of complex carbohydrates in the way of foods as grown: vegetables, fruits, grains, and legumes
2. plenty of food products made with little or no processing, such as whole grain pasta and whole grain cereals; less of food products that have been significantly processed or "predigested," such as white flour and precooked cereals
3. no sugar, fat, or salt and no foods made with sugar, fat, or salt
4. restricted choices of meat, fruit, and dairy products.*

*Meat and dairy products are restricted in order to control the amounts of fat and cholesterol in your diet. Dietary cholesterol needs to be controlled because it is strongly linked to early death from heart attack and other degenerative diseases. It can be argued that the fatlike substance cholesterol does not contribute to overweight. Nevertheless, it is closely allied to the fat in animal products (you can hardly eat one without the other) and is strongly linked to killer diseases. Dietary salt, too, is controlled largely because of the health benefits this achieves. As

Foods that are within the Live Longer Now diet are what I call "longevity foods." I call other foods "problem foods" because I feel they truly are problems. (There is a detailed discussion of longevity foods and how to get them in Chapter 5.)

Figure 1.1 compares the longevity native-style diet with the average American diet and the dietary goals for Americans recommended by the U.S. Senate's Select Committee on Nutrition. It is obvious from the figure that the native-style diet is drastically different from the average American diet. The Senate's recommended diet also alters the average American diet considerably.

Don't let the high level of complex carbohydrates in the native-style diet worry you. You really can't get too much of these vegetables, fruits, grains, and legumes. Actually, the Senate's recommended level of carbohydrates is almost 60 percent (43 percent from complex carbohydrates and 15 percent from sugar, which is merely a predigested complex carbohydrate), not far from the native diet level of 78 percent.

Don't worry about the low fat content in the native diet either. Your body can make all the fat it needs from the complex carbohydrates you eat. The minimum daily levels of dietary fat required by the body can be measured in drops and are far less than the 10 percent that occurs naturally in the native diet.

You may have noticed that I use the term native-style diet or native diet interchangeably with longevity diet and that I have interchanged this term with Live Longer Now diet. Although the terms have grown from different usages, they are completely interchangeable. This interchangeability is formalized in the diagram on page 17. In this book they all mean the same food and the same style of eating.

Quick Weight Loss

How fast can a person lose weight? That depends a little on the person and a lot on whether the weight being lost is fat or simply water.

Dr. Leonard Berman said recently in a comprehensive review in the *Journal of the American Medical Association:* "There is now strong evidence that [the killer disease hypertension] can be eradicated by the adoption of a diet that contains no more than 2 grams of salt per day." The Live Longer Now diet and native-style diets in general fall safely within this limit.

Average American Diet	Diet Recommended by the U.S. Senate's Nutrition Committee	Longevity Native-Style Diet
25% Sugar	15% Sugar	10% Fat
		12% Protein
42% Fat	30% Fat	78% Complex Carbohydrates
	12% Protein	
12% Protein	43% Complex Carbohydrates	
21% Complex Carbohydrates		

Figure 1.1. Comparison of Longevity Native-Style Diet with the Average American Diet and the Recommended Diet of the U.S. Senate's Nutrition Committee.

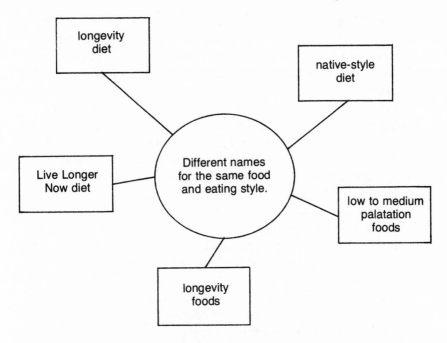

You can easily lose weight by losing fluids from your body. Virtually anyone can lose several pounds of body weight in that manner in a single day. On a hot day a long-distance runner in Arizona can lose ten pounds in an hour or two. Almost every bit of that loss is from water lost through perspiration and water lost through the mouth from the rapid breathing involved in running. The runner's body fat has changed very little in comparison.

Every diet program that claims to produce rapid large weight loss is doing one of two things: lying or creating a loss of body water. Neither of these things is good. Lying is reprehensible, and losing body water is irrelevant and potentially dangerous to your health. You don't need to lose water; you need to lose fat.

The real question is: How fast can you lose fat? On a complete starvation fast the average dieter can lose about a half pound of fat per day; no more. Body fat is such a superefficient energy storer that a mere half pound of it will power your body all day and all night. So, if you eat no food at all, that's how much fat your body will use up in order to operate for one whole day.

Thus, ½ pound of fat per day amounts to just under 4 pounds of fat per week. For the average dieter, this is the fastest rate of weight loss possible under the most extreme situation: starvation. Starvation is not the answer, however. Starvation fasts can be dangerous, can deplete your body of critical nutrients, and can leave you with excessively sagging skin.

Your Live Longer Now program produces the optimum speed of losing weight: a little more than one pound of weight loss a week in the beginning of your program tapering to a little less than a pound a week as you approach your goal. For the average dieter this level of weight loss can be achieved by engaging in a little extra physical activity and reducing caloric intake by about 25 percent.

In the first ten days or two weeks the Live Longer Now program will probably cause you to lose a large amount of weight in unavoidable water loss, as much as a pound a day. From that point on, the program settles into an optimum weight loss of approximately one pound a week.

The Live Longer Now quick-weight-loss program provides the quickest possible weight loss consistent with good health. What is equally important, it gives the quickest possible weight loss consistent with long-term success.

Complications of Overweight

I don't like scare tactics, and I don't think many people are influenced by them. But I want to talk about some scary things, some diseases, associated with excess fatness. My desire is not to scare but to inform. You may as well know that losing weight brings you benefits beyond simply looking better and feeling better. It helps you live a longer life free of disease.

You should know that if you are excessively fat you have a much greater risk of dying suddenly from heart attack than if you are at your best weight. If you are obese, your chances are much greater of developing angina pectoris, the intense chest pains that heart patients frequently suffer. And the greater your fatness, the worse your chances on both counts.

Overweight, your chances of getting high blood pressure are as much as five times greater than average, and your chances of dying from hypertensive heart disease or stroke are correspondingly greater. Your chances of developing diabetes are 300 percent of normal, as is your chance of developing gall bladder disease. Your risk of death from kidney failure is 200 percent of normal.

If you have to have surgery for one of these conditions, your risks are great. Your surgeon will have to use a larger than normal incision, and will have to cut through a thick layer of hindering fat to get at his target. He will have to tie off many more blood vessels and will have to do much more work to keep the incision open. At every step in suturing the incision, your surgeon will have to unstick fat from his sutures. All in all, you will be under anesthesia longer than a lean person will; and because your breathing may be seriously impaired by your overweight, the possibility of respiratory failure is greater. Even after the surgery, your recovery is still in doubt. You have a much increased chance of wound infection, reopening of the wound, and blood clotting.

Finally, if you are a woman, your fatness will be passed along to your baby. The troubles you now have will become those of your offspring.

It is depressing to dwell on the complications of excessive fatness. I prefer not to dwell on them. I prefer to recognize the complications but focus on other things: losing weight, feeling good, and living a long, healthy life.

What about Children and Teenagers?

Obesity frequently begins in childhood: as early as the first year, or as late as the teen-age years. Once a youth becomes obese, cellular changes in adipose tissue may occur that may make it extremely difficult to control obesity in later life. The prevention of youthful obesity is absolutely essential to the prevention of adult obesity.

The Live Longer Now program may be used for children and teen-agers as well as for adults. It may be used as a reducing program for the overweight child or teen-ager as well as a prevention program for the normal-weight child or teen-ager. The program provides an adequate supply of all the vitamins and minerals needed by growing children. Protein intake is about the same, in overall amounts, as the protein intake of the average American today. The type of protein is different, consisting largely of vegetable protein rather than the animal protein that makes up the usual American diet; in my view a distinct advantage.

This program is meant to be lifelong. It provides a natural diet that is as close to an "optimal human diet" as we know how to get at this time, a good diet for the young to become acquainted with. The usefulness of the diet in preventing heart disease and stroke is also of importance to the young, because it is now known that the vessel disease that leads to heart attacks and strokes in later life actually has its beginnings in childhood. Therefore it is in childhood that prevention should begin.

Are You Ready for Longevity Eating?

Some weight-loss programs are much easier than the Live Longer Now program. But these programs do not work. The Live Longer Now program is the easiest weight-loss program that actually works.

The program is hard in some ways and easy in others. It is hard because there is learning involved. You have to learn how to tell the difference between longevity foods and other foods, how to prepare longevity foods, and how to deal with a world centered on nonlongevity foods. It is easy because once you have accommodated yourself to longevity eating, weight loss is sure and pleasant. You will feel adequately nourished and you'll never feel particularly hungry.

Anyone can adopt the Live Longer Now program. Literally hundreds of thousands of people have. And many of those who have, haven't been overweight. Their interest was purely their own good health.

If you are ready to commit yourself to a new life style and are willing to learn about foods and about yourself, you can expect to be successful in the Live Longer Now program. If you're only mildly interested in permanent weight loss or are not ready to commit yourself to change, your chances of success are much smaller. In that case I would rather you wait to begin the program until you have put more thought into it and are mentally prepared for it.

To test your readiness to begin the program, I have prepared a

Readiness Test for you (see below). Look the test over and answer the questions. If you can answer yes to all six questions, you are ready to go. Don't waste any time. Get started now.

If you answer no to any of the questions, you should probably wait a while before you start the program. But you will get significant benefit by reading Chapter 11.

If you answered no to a question, think about your reasons for doing so. Can you foresee circumstances under which you would change your answer to yes? Can you make those circumstances occur? Take the Readiness Test again in a few weeks; you may be surprised to find that you have changed your thinking and are ready to begin the program in earnest.

READINESS TEST

	Yes	No
1. Are you willing to learn and apply facts about food composition?	☐	☐
2. Are you willing to keep records of your food habits?	☐	☐
3. Are you willing to set two weeks aside before you begin your weight-losing program for a period of learning and adaptation?	☐	☐
4. Are you willing to change the kinds of food you eat?	☐	☐
5. Are you willing to exercise?	☐	☐
6. Are you looking for permanent weight loss?	☐	☐

CHAPTER 2

How the Live Longer Now Quick Weight-Loss Program Works

Your goal is to lose pounds and achieve an ideal body weight as quickly as possible consistent with good health and lasting success. The Live Longer Now Quick Weight-Loss program is a scientifically engineered step-by-step process to get you to your goal.

Two basic programs are involved: a food program and an activity program. Each is important to your goal and each helps the other to achieve that goal.

By acting as a mild appetite suppressant, physical activity helps make the food program a success. And the food program, by supplying a rich source of excellent nutrients, makes physical activity more fun and easier to do. Figure 2.1 shows the mutually supportive role the food program and the activity program play in weight loss and the chapters in which each program is discussed.

The activity program involves a new concept called "roving," the easiest exercise a human being can perform, and the most beneficial. This program can be started with little preparation or fanfare. Simply read Chapters 3 and 4 and begin.

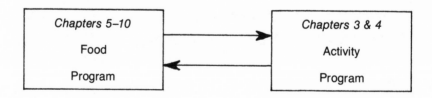

Figure 2.1. Live Longer Now Quick Weight-Loss Program

The food program is more involved. Food habits and practices are so complex in our society that a substantial amount of learning and unlearning are needed. The food program is contained in Chapters 5 through 10.

Figure 2.2 shows the three major phases of the food program. Phase 1, the start-up phase, takes a little more than two weeks to accomplish and is the most complicated of the phases. It's where you learn everything you have to learn in order to accomplish the next two phases. Phase 2, the weight-losing phase, takes as long as is necessary to reach your weight-loss goal. Typically this is a matter of months if you lose at the proper rate: not so fast as to gain it all back, and not so slow as to be discouraging. Phase 3, long-term maintenance, is a lifelong process in which you practice the simple principles of the Live Longer Now program so as to remain slim and healthy.

Let's begin with the start-up phase, where all the new ideas are

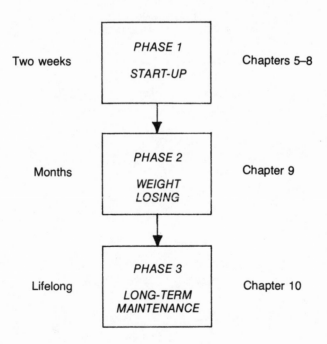

Figure 2.2. The Food Program

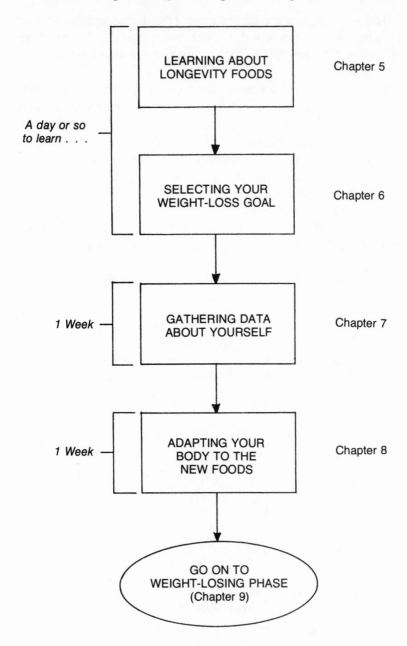

Figure 2.3. Start-Up Phase

introduced. Figure 2.3 shows what you will be doing during the start-up phase.

First, you will spend a day or so in reading and reflection in order to learn what you need to know about longevity foods (what they are, how to shop for them, and how to prepare them) and to establish your goal weight, the target you will strive for as you lose weight. Next, you will take a week to gather data about yourself (your eating and your activity habits) and experiment a little with longevity foods. Last, you will spend a week *adapting your body* to longevity foods. This important process is done before the weight-losing phase begins.

The food program involves recordkeeping, quite a lot of it at first. You will be keeping journals, making detailed plans, and checking your progress. If this seems like a lot of work, relax. You will be given a step-by-step guide through each thing to be done. By the time the start-up phase is finished, you will have completed all recordkeeping except for charting your progress. And when you achieve your goal weight, you can even dispense with that. Figure 2.4 shows the recordkeeping required and how it diminishes as you progress.

DATA GATHERING
Eating Journal
Activities Journal

PLANNING
Meal Plan
Action Plan

KEEPING TRACK OF PROGRESS
FLAB Control Cards
Score Chart

| | | |

KEEPING TRACK OF PROGRESS
FLAB Control Cards
Score Chart

No formal recordkeeping needed!

START-UP PHASE   WEIGHT-LOSING PHASE   LONG-TERM MAINTENANCE PHASE

Figure 2.4. Recordkeeping Required

The Six Steps to Weight Loss

To sum up: There are six steps to the Live Longer Now Weight-Loss program. These steps are as follows:

1. Begin Exercise Program (read Chapters 3 and 4).
2. Learn about Longevity Foods (read Chapter 5).
3. Select Your Goal Weight (read Chapter 6).
4. Gather Data on Yourself (read Chapter 7).
5. Adapt to Longevity Eating (read Chapter 8).
6. Begin Weight-Losing Program (read Chapter 9).

These six steps will take you to the heart of the program. Time will take you from there to your goal.

If You Want a Faster Start

The six-step process takes time. As mentioned, it takes a little more than fourteen days before you actually begin the weight-losing program. The natural question is: Can the process be speeded up? Can I start losing weight immediately?

The answer is yes, with qualifications. All you need is a knowledge of longevity foods and an idea of how to apply that knowledge to begin losing weight. The six-step process provides a carefully thought out approach to longevity eating. But if you are the type who prefers to race ahead with your own approach, by all means do so.

Read Chapters 3, 4, and 5 first. They will tell you the basic facts. If after reading Chapter 5 on longevity foods you agree the subject is complex and you need ideas on how to proceed, read Chapters 6, 7, and 8 to give you insightful ideas. Once you feel you have enough facts and know how to proceed, simply begin. If you feel that your approach is not working as well as you would like it to, you always have the six-step process as a sure-fire approach to fall back on.

CHAPTER 3

Roving

There is one basic reason you or anyone else concerned about weight loss should be interested in activity: It makes losing weight easier. Weight loss works best when coupled with physical activity. And the best form of physical activity is a form called "roving." Roving involves getting around on your own two feet; it is the simplest, most natural form of exercise a human being can take. Before talking about roving in particular, let's talk about physical activity in general, and why it is important to you.

Food and Energy

You eat food because your body needs it for energy. Your body also needs food for some of the body-building chemicals it must have, but most of your food goes for energy. All the things you do—walking, bending, carrying, lifting, and even breathing—take energy, and this energy is supplied by the food you eat. Even the chemical processes that go on inside your body cells use energy, which must come from food.

The reason scientists talk about the calories in food is that calories measure how much energy food has. A 10-calorie cracker has only one-third as much energy as a 30-calorie apple, for example. And a candy bar has a great deal of energy, as we all know, because it has so many calories.

The calorie is a scientific concept. It is a measure of how much energy is contained in a substance. A calorie of energy is a lot of energy. It is enough energy to raise the temperature of a quart of water about 2 degrees Fahrenheit. If applied right, 100 calories could bring a quart of water to a rolling boil. Yet people eat thousands of calories every day and don't even get singed.

Our bodies are wonderfully efficient mechanisms. If we eat any quantity of food, no matter how much, our bodies process every bit of it and extract out of it every scrap of energy it has to offer. If we don't use up all this energy by activities like walking, bending, lifting, and breathing, or by chemical processes like digestion, protein making, and enzyme action, we just store the extra energy away for a rainy day. We store it as a high-energy substance, fat. And the more fat we store away (for rainy days that never come), the fatter our bodies become.

Exercise obviously has the potential for helping us lose weight because as we use up extra energy roving, swimming, jumping rope, and the like, there is that much less energy to be stored away in the form of fat. But exercise does far more than use up extra calories. If it did only that, perhaps it could be dispensed with in a weight-loss program. It can't be dispensed with because it does other, critical things.

Food and Activity

Scientific opinion is often slower to reflect the truth than popular opinion is. This has happened repeatedly in the scientific investigation of overweight. One instance has to do with overweight and activity.

Popular opinion has held for years that overweight is closely related to inactivity. Fat farms have always used increased physical activity to slim people down, whereas the farmer has done the opposite to fatten his animals. If the farmer puts his pig in a small pen with no room to move around, the pig gains weight rapidly.

Scientific opinion had not really grasped this truth prior to 1954. It had been thought that changes in activity would always be accompanied by a compensating change in food eaten. If one were to exercise an overweight animal (or person), it was believed that there would simply be a compensating increase in food intake.

In 1954 Jean Mayer and his associates at the Harvard School of Public Health destroyed this myth. Dr. Mayer exercised laboratory rats on a treadmill, and at the same time he carefully measured the food these rats consumed. What he found surprised the experts, even though it may not have come as a surprise to the pig farmer.

The results of Dr. Mayer's experiment are shown in Figure 3.1, which shows the amount of food these animals ate corresponding to the level of exercise they were forced to undergo. The surprise was that they ate the least food when they exercised for an hour a day. They did not eat the least food when they were completely inactive, as many scientists would have guessed. In fact, below an hour a day's exercise, the animals ate increasingly more food. With no exercise, the animals ate as much food as they did with two hours of daily exercise.

Dr. Mayer also kept track of the animals' body weights. Not surprisingly, he found that animals who were exercised an hour or more a day maintained a normal body weight while those who were exercised less than an hour a day became increasingly overweight. At no exercise at all the animals became obese, 33 percent over their normal body weight. (This would be equivalent to a 150-pound man becoming 50 pounds overweight.)

Dr. Mayer's experiment showed that the appetite mechanism in

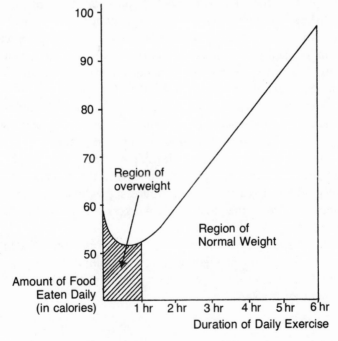

Figure 3.1. Daily Food Intake Versus Amount of Daily Exercise

these animals worked well when the animals exercised, but failed when they did not. It also showed that there is a *critical exercise level* (1 hour), below which these animals tended to overweight and above which overweight was absent.

In their natural state rats expend energy in their continual quest for food. Under these conditions rats will naturally and automatically exceed the critical exercise level that separates overweight from normal weight. Obese rats are not found in nature.

It is likely that primitive humans were in pretty much the same boat. In their quest for food and shelter, their activity level was probably fairly high—well above whatever the corresponding critical level in humans is. This situation probably prevailed in most parts of the world until the advent of the machine age.

When machine power began to replace muscle power, all this changed. Today in the United States our lives are mainly sedentary. Our jobs are largely sedentary (sit-down jobs), and our home lives are sedentary too. We sit all day at the office and come home to plop down on the sofa, exhausted from sitting all day. We have cars to get us to work, elevators and escalators to bypass stairways, and heated offices to keep our bodies from having to generate their own heat. We have electric can openers, electric toothbrushes, and pop-top cans. Increasingly the favorite American sport is football, watched on TV from an easy chair, beer glass in hand. No wonder America has become the overweight capital of the world.

It is common knowledge that exercise is important in weight-loss programs, for humans and animals both. Dr. Mayer showed how it works in rats. He also showed how it works in people.

Dr. Mayer investigated the relationship between body weight and level of activity in the workplace for people in India. This relationship is shown in Figure 3.2. The figure shows that workers with sedentary jobs weigh the most, while workers with medium-activity jobs weigh the least.

Figure 3.3 shows the amount of food these workers eat. Sedentary workers eat more food than light workers, medium workers, or heavy workers. Only workers with very heavy activity jobs eat more food than sedentary workers.

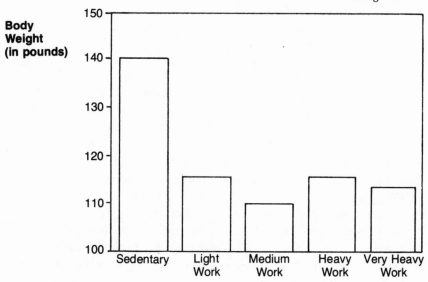

Body Weight (in pounds)

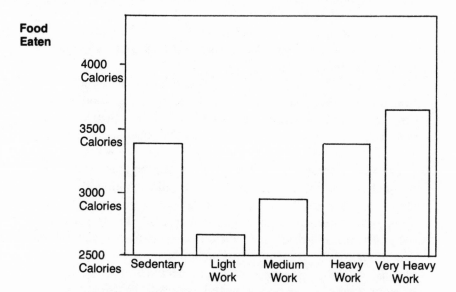

Food Eaten

Figure 3.2. Body Weight Versus Activity Level for Working People in India

Figure 3.3 Amount of Food Eaten Versus Activity Level for Working People in India

Exercise and Appetite

It is striking that, up to a point, both animals and humans eat less food as they engage in more exercise. What this means is that exercise has some controlling influence on appetite.

Appetite, the desire to eat, depends on a number of things. For example, it depends on the fullness of the stomach, the blood sugar level, and the level of circulating hormones such as insulin. These things are inside the body. Appetite also depends on things outside the body: the attractiveness of food, food palatability, and the presence of other food cues. In humans, appetite depends on emotional factors as well. Many people have a desire to eat as a response to pressure, tension, or repressed feelings. Others lose their desire to eat under the same conditions.

Clearly, appetite is complex, involving many things. But overriding this complexity is the simple fact that exercise can reduce appetite. How does exercise do this?

In the opening pages of this book we discussed the satiety center in the brain. As we saw, the satiety center is probably not working well in obese people.

One reason for the failure of the satiety center is thought to be related to the abnormally high level of insulin in the blood of obese people. Abnormal insulin levels directly affect the satiety center and may well account for its failure to warn the obese person to stop eating.

The more overweight an individual is, and the longer the excess weight has been present, the greater the insulin abnormality. Americans as a group are overweight. And American insulin levels, as a group, are abnormally high and react abnormally to sugar loading.

In 1970 Bjorntorp, of the University of Gothenburg, showed that exercise normalizes the blood insulin of obese people. In his experiment Bjorntorp had severely overweight people exercise for a period of eight weeks. These people were instructed to eat freely of their normal foods. At the end of the eight-week period their insulin levels were measured and compared with the levels at the start of the experiment. The insulin levels at the end were only half of what they

were at the beginning. Other parameters, such as blood sugar, cholesterol, and triglycerides, showed little change. But the change in
insulin was consistent and dramatic.

Basal Metabolism

Whether you feel energetic or not, your body uses energy. Even
when you are flat on your back in bed, resting and relaxing, your
body uses energy, lots of it, to keep all the bodily processes going.
The activities you engage in—like washing the car, mopping the
floor, or walking to work—use energy over and above that required
to maintain your body.

The rate at which you use energy while you are lying down resting
and relaxed is called your Basal Metabolic Rate (BMR). This rate of
energy usage theoretically goes on all day and all night, no matter
what else you do. It is the idle speed of your body. Whatever else you
do simply adds energy on top of your BMR.

Everyone's BMR is different. Some people have efficient bodies.
Their bodies don't require much energy to idle, and so their BMR is
low. But some people's bodies idle at a roar. Their BMR is high.

It is common for overweight people to have a low BMR. This
means that it doesn't take much energy to run their bodily processes.
But it also means that it doesn't take much food either. This is a
common problem with overweight people: A little food is enough to
handle their energy needs, and a bit more than a little will cause them
to gain weight.

Here again, exercise helps. Of course exercise helps to use up
calories directly. We all know that. But what is not commonly known
is that exercise can actually increase your BMR for many hours after
you have stopped exercising. Thus, exercise helps use calories while
you are exercising, but by increasing your BMR, exercise also uses
calories after you've stopped exercising.

Dr. U. D. Register at Loma Linda University measured the BMR
of obese people after exercise. Dr. Register had his patients run on a
treadmill until they had used up 100 calories. He found that following
this exercise, the BMRs of these patients increased by 10 to 15
percent and remained at the higher rate for 24 hours. Thus these

people used at least another 200 calories, as a result of the higher BMR, after the exercise was over. This means that the effect of this exercise was tripled by the effect on the BMR.

Dr. Register was not the first to measure the effect of exercise on the BMR. As early as 1963 the aftereffects of exercise on the BMR were noted by Gray and deVries, who reported their study of two individuals whose BMR was increased after exercise so that 53 calories were used up in the 6 hours following a 45-minute exercise session. Other researchers have confirmed these results.

The Activity Habits of Overweight People

The noted physician Albert Stunkard has spent many years at Stanford studying overweight people. An important part of his studies concerns the activity habits of obese people. Assuming that one's activity level is pretty much reflected by the distance one walks each day—at work, at home, and at play—Dr. Stunkard strapped pedometers on obese and normal-weight people to see how they differed. A pedometer is a small device about the size of a stopwatch; it can be connected to your belt and worn while you are engaged in your normal activities. It keeps track of how far you've walked during the day; you simply read out your distance each night before you retire.

Dr. Stunkard found that normal-weight women walked about 4.5 miles per day, while obese women walked much less: only 1.5 miles per day.

He also found that activity corresponded most closely to cultural expectations. Obese girls at camp, for example, averaged as much distance walked as normal-weight girls. And at camp obese girls ate less than usual and lost weight, whereas normal-weight girls ate more than usual and gained weight.

On a job that demands activity, an obese person can and will muster the wherewithal to get the job done. Nowhere is this more clear than for men undergoing military basic training. In a survey of obese men who had completed a relatively mild basic training, Stunkard found that all the men had lost weight. The weight loss averaged 20 pounds, with some men losing as much as 30 pounds.

Moreover, the men commented that the weight loss had come painlessly. They had been free to eat as much as they wanted, and did so.

All of this shows that the activity habits of overweight people, while perhaps reduced compared with normal-weight people, are nevertheless more culturally related than anything else. When the culture demands it—at camp, at military training, or on the job—overweight people can do it.

Exercise and Health

Your main interest in exercise will no doubt be to make losing weight easier. But you shouldn't ignore the importance of exercise to your general health. Regular exercise promotes health and provides protection from disease.

Exercise Against Disease

Heart disease and other degenerative diseases are the most prominent causes of death in America. Anything that will blunt the life-shortening effect of these diseases is to be welcomed. Exercise does this.

Dr. Charles W. Frank and associates studied 55,000 men enrolled in the Health Insurance Plan of Greater New York. They found that among people in this plan who subsequently had a heart attack, inactive people were far more likely than active people to suffer a fatal or severe attack. His study showed that if you had a heart attack and were in the most active group, your chances of dying from the attack were only a third of what they would be if you were in the least active group. And your chances of having a serious but nonfatal attack were less than half what they would be if you were less active.

Ralph Paffenbarger of the California Department of Health studied longshoremen in San Francisco, comparing high-energy jobs with low-energy jobs. Paffenbarger not only found that people in the high-energy jobs had lower death rates from heart disease, he also demonstrated that it was the job itself that caused the death rates to be lower. That is, he showed that, among longshoremen, it was not a matter of healthier, stronger people taking the hard jobs while sickly, heart-disease-prone people took softer jobs. The people were statistically the same—only the jobs differed. And the hard, high-energy jobs provided protection from heart attack.

Bodily Changes

Exercise changes things in the body. These changes are good changes, reflecting a better ability to handle blood flow, use oxygen, and use body fat.

Many researchers have noticed and reported on changes that take place when people exercise. For example, John Hanson at the University of Vermont tested seven middle-aged sedentary people, then placed them on an exercise program for half a year. The exercise was for an hour a day, three days a week, and consisted of warm-up, jogging, paddleball, and other enjoyable activities. At the end of the program the participants were retested. Dr. Hanson found that the resting heart rate of his subjects had decreased from an average of 81 to an average of 65. A lower heart rate means the heart is pumping blood more efficiently. (In fact, the average participant was saving over 20,000 heartbeats a day because of this efficiency.) Dr. Hanson also found that the average subject was able to utilize 17 percent more of the oxygen breathed in during an exercise bout, indicating a better efficiency in both delivery of oxygen and incorporation of oxygen into the body's cells. He also found that the total volume of blood carried in the body had increased in these people.

Jack Wilmore of the University of Arizona also investigated the physiological effects of exercise on people. In a three-month study involving 44 people on a simple exercise program, Dr. Wilmore found changes in heart and oxygen parameters, and he also found that whole body composition was altered. The body's pool of fat had decreased an average of 18 percent, and the body's lean mass had increased by 1 percent.

General Complaints

Aside from the benefits of protection from heart disease and improvement in bodily parameters, exercise also just plain makes you feel better. Figure 3.4 is a list of the general complaints most

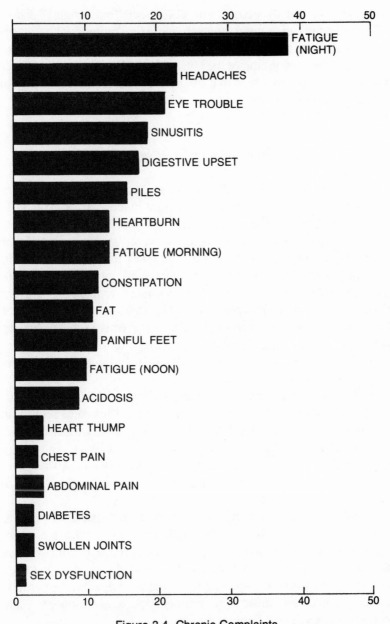

Figure 3.4. Chronic Complaints.
From *Physiological Effects of Exercise in Adults* by Thomas K. Cureton (1969). Courtesy of
Charles C. Thomas, Publisher, Springfield, Illinois.

frequently voiced by people who don't feel "quite right." Complaints like fatigue or upset stomach may seem minor but are important. They make the difference between feeling great and feeling out of sorts. Thomas Cureton of the University of Illinois Fitness Center found that people involved in a fitness program are far less likely to report these chronic complaints than other people.

Looking Good and Feeling Good

In helping you lose weight, exercise helps you become more attractive. And more attractive in the right places. Dr. Melvin Williams, director of the Human Performance Laboratory at Old Dominion University, has considered the question of "spot reducing," that is, getting rid of ugly bulges. Everyone tends to carry excess fat in favorite places. And these are the most unsightly places and often the hardest places to trim down. Dr. Williams summarizes current thought on exercise and spot reducing by stating that "reduction of body fat in body areas is most likely to occur where fat deposits are the most conspicuous, regardless of the exercise format." With diet alone, the ugly bulges may be the last to go. But with exercise they are the first to go.

Activity is closely related to the psychological feeling of well-being. Duddleston and Bennion studied weight loss and activity in twelve obese college coeds. They placed some of the women on a diet and exercise program and some on a diet program only. Those who combined diet and exercise lost more in the twelve-week study and also exhibited "greater feelings of physical well-being" and "a more positive mental attitude."

Czechoslovakia has started a national effort to stem its postwar outbreak of obesity. Overweight people from all over the nation are being placed on either a diet program or a diet program with exercise added. The psychological benefits of the added program have been confirmed by psychological testing of the participants. Test results have revealed that those who exercise are better motivated and experience much less depression.

The effect of activity on mental health has been so striking that exercise is now being used as therapy for mental illness by a number of researchers. Dr. Robert Brown of the University of Virginia has used running as therapy for over 2000 patients, and states: "I have demonstrated to my satisfaction that athletic-type training will reduce both anxiety and depression at the highly significant level."

Roving: The Live Longer Now Way to Exercise

The human form of locomotion is unique among mammals. Only the human being moves about in an upright posture on two legs, with a stride and gait as smooth and liquid at a high rate of speed as it is at a slow amble.

Anthropologists tell us that humans acquired their unique form of travel over a million years ago. And for the last million years they have hunted, played, built, and traveled—at slow speed and fast speed—on two legs.

Human beings are so incredibly adapted to two-legged locomotion that fantastic feats of endurance and long-distance travel have been recorded by people. Mensen Ernst of Norway, for instance, holds the world's record for long-distance travel, having covered nearly 100 miles a day, on foot, for nearly two months—5500 miles in all. In fact, humans are as good as, and perhaps superior to, all other land animals in long-distance travel.

I say these things for one purpose—to let you know that moving around on your two legs is an activity to which you are ideally suited, no matter who you are.* The largest muscles in your body are in your legs. Exercising these muscles will bring faster changes in your body chemistry and makeup than exercising any other muscle group.

Anyone can walk. Anyone can learn to jog. Roving is the use of walking, jogging, or both to gain control over your physical condition.

The key concept behind roving is distance. Time is not the point. Speed is not the point. Distance is the point.

When a primitive man traveled long distances, his object was to get from here to there. He could do it well. He set a pace dictated by how he felt at the moment. He might jog, he might run, or he might walk.

---

*This applies to all nonhandicapped individuals. Handicapped individuals still need activity like everyone else, and can get it in other ways: swimming, wheelchair basketball, etc.

He experienced the land and objects through which he moved, and he experienced the reward of arriving at his destination at the end.

Roving is like this. You dictate your pace by how you feel: your desires and your physical condition. You walk, you jog, or you run as your ability and desires dictate. You cover distance from here to there, and you don't concern yourself with time or pace. You see the land and objects through which you move, and you are rewarded by arriving at your destination.

You may begin roving right now. You don't have to be in shape and you don't need special equipment. You can do it any time of year and any time of the day. Here is how you start:

1. Select a distance to rove and a pleasant route to follow. In the beginning choose a distance that will take you about 20 to 30 minutes to accomplish.
2. If you are unconditioned,* do not run or jog for the first 6 weeks. Simply walk. At the end of 6 weeks, you may begin to jog. Read Chapter 4 on running and jogging.
3. Rove a minimum of 5 days per week, selecting new roving routes, from time to time, for variety.
4. Increase your distance and your pace whenever you are ready. At the end of 6 weeks, you should be roving approximately an hour per day at a pace of 4 miles per hour.

These simple rules are easy to follow. You can begin now.

Roving requires one piece of equipment: a good pair of shoes. Comfortable street shoes with a soft sole may be good enough at first. But sooner or later you will want to invest in truly excellent footwear. Without question the best shoes for walking, jogging, or running are the runners' shoes sold at sporting goods stores. They are called "training flats" by professionals (meaning that runners use them in their long-distance training runs). Many outstanding brands are available. I recommend Nike, Adidas, or New Balance. Take it from me, a runner's shoe is the most comfortable shoe you'll ever own. The ultra soft and thickly padded sole will make roving a dream.

---

*Unless you have engaged in regular physical activity of an endurance nature at least 3 days per week for the previous 6 weeks, you should assume you are unconditioned.

CHAPTER 4

Jogging and Running

This chapter will try to convince you that you should learn to jog or run. And it will provide you with guidelines that will help you learn—safely and enjoyably.

There was a time in your life when you were fit. Your body obeyed your commands to move and explore the world around you. You woke each morning fresh and alive, like a healthy animal. Sounds, sights, and smells were sharp and clear. Your energy was limitless.

Can those days of fitness be recovered? Yes they can. Learning to jog or run is the way to do it.

Learning is easier today than it was a few years ago because there are so many people already running. The psychological barrier of being the only person doing it is gone. According to Dr. John Cantwell of the President's Council on Physical Fitness, over 10 percent of the people in our country run regularly. That's 22 million people to keep you company.

Many of these people have discovered what I discovered: Running is its own reward. I began running for physical health, but I continued running for the ineffable experience it provides. Many people have written about "runner's high." But these words can't begin to describe the marvelous feeling of well-being that running can bring, a feeling that lasts all day and enhances every other endeavor.

Dr. George Sheehan says it this way: "What lies beyond fitness-for-muscle is the 'third wind.' The third wind is psychological, unlike the second wind which is physical. When I hit my third wind, I see myself not as an individual, but as part of the universe."

The Tarahumara Indians have evolved a national sport involving long-distance running. Their social life revolves around this sport, and entire villages take part in it. Participants run for incredibly long times without stopping. Scores of miles and many hours pass before a game ends.

Why do these people do it? What's in it for them? Perhaps they have discovered what I discovered: The run is the reward.

According to an article on these Indians in the *Journal of the American Medical Association*, the Tarahumarans are characterized by their quiet dignity, respect for others, good humor among themselves, and helpfulness to strangers. Intergroup or interpersonal violence is unknown, as is divorce and alcoholism (in spite of the availability of alcohol). As W. E. Connor found, obesity, high blood pressure, and heart disease are also unknown among the Tarahumarans. Thus, whatever the reason for their running, it's worth doing.

Would you feel self-conscious about running at your present weight? Welcome to the crowd. Many people start running solely because of a weight problem. And most are self-conscious in the beginning. Just realize that literally millions of people have been able to overcome these feelings, and 10 or 50 or 75 pounds later, they are glad they did.

Age need be no barrier, either. Dr. Cantwell of the President's Council of Physical Fitness tells of people in their 60s who take up running for the first time and are running marathon races (over 26 miles) in their 70s. I know of many examples personally, including a 90-year-old great-grandmother who took up running at 81 years of age. She took up running (together with the Live Longer Now diet) as therapy for a severe heart condition and other degenerative ailments. It worked. At ages 85, 86, and 87, she won gold medals in the Senior Olympics in the mile and half mile races in her age category.

It is not my desire to turn you into a Tarahumara Indian or a racing athlete. I simply want to awaken in you the knowledge that you *can* learn to run, and if you do learn, you will be rewarded.

Medical Clearance

Before you begin a roving program that involves jogging or running, you must get a go-ahead from your family doctor. By completing a medical history, a detailed physical exam, and laboratory tests involving an EKG and blood chemistries, a doctor can determine whether there are reasons for not exercising.

Only an expert can tell you if you have a condition that would make unsupervised activity dangerous. For the vast majority of us, there is no danger in a gradual, progressive exercise program. But for that rare individual, a danger can exist. In particular, don't begin an unsupervised exercise program if you know that you have any of these conditions: angina pectoris, recent heart attack, disease of the heart valves, congenital heart disease, enlarged heart due to hypertension, severe irregularities of the heartbeat needing medication, uncontrolled diabetes, or other conditions needing close medical supervision.

Beginning to Run

If there is one commandment that stands out above all others when you are a beginning runner, it is this: Take it slow. There is no hurry. You have spent years not running, and you should be willing to spend at least a little time in becoming a runner.

Don't begin running if you have not read page 40 on how to start roving. If you are "conditioned," or have completed six weeks of preparatory roving as described there, then you are ready to begin running.

Begin running by mixing walking and jogging in what is known as "scout pace." Alternate walking with very easy jogging: 25 paces walking alternated with 25 paces jogging. In time you will be able to increase the amount of jogging you do and decrease the amount of walking, until finally you are jogging all the time. How long this takes depends on your capabilities and will vary between 1 and 4 weeks.

Pace

Pace may be the key to enjoyable running. Runners often think of pace in terms of minutes per mile. If you were to ask a runner at what pace he does his training, he might say something like "an eight-minute-mile pace." The runner thinks of pace as speed: distance and time.

I prefer to think of pace the way George Sheehan does: in terms of the personal effort the running requires. Thus pace is best thought of in terms like very easy, easy, comfortable, somewhat hard, hard, or very hard.

In running, whether you are inexperienced or an old pro, your pace can always be the same. Set your pace at "comfortable" and enjoy your rove. Avoid a hard pace. Use Oregon track coach Bill Bowerman's talk test: Can you carry on a conversation during your rove without becoming breathless? If so, your pace is set in the comfort range and is the right pace for you.

Your Heart Rate

A good indicator of your pace is your heartbeat. The faster your heart beats during a rove, the harder your pace is. You can determine how fast your heart is beating by simply stopping to take your pulse.

If you are a beginning runner, it is extremely important to take your pulse in the middle and at the end of every rove. Your pulse rate will notify you if you are exceeding your capabilities and will also tell you if you are loafing too much and taking it too easy.

To take your pulse, you need a watch with a secondhand or a digital watch that reads out seconds. Take your pulse by feeling the pulsations in your throat at either side of your Adam's apple or by feeling the pulse at your wrist like the nurses on television do it. Once in the middle of your rove and once at the end, stop and immediately count how many pulses you get in *10 seconds*.

Use this 10-second count to see if your pace is a "comfortable" pace as far as your heart is concerned. A comfortable pulse depends on your age. There is an easy way to determine what a comfortable 10-second pulse should be for you. Simply subtract one-tenth of your age from 24. This is your comfortable 10-second pulse. Table 4.1 will do the math for you, if you prefer.

Your comfortable 10-second pulse is your "target heart rate," that is, the ideal rate for your heart to beat during a rove. Your target heart rate (it is commonly abbreviated THR) will stay the same even as you get in better and better shape. As your condition improves, you'll just be able to go farther and faster without getting out of the comfortable range.

Table 4.1 shows THRs for different ages. Find your THR right now, and write it down someplace. This is an important number for you. Take your 10-second pulse twice in each rove, and compare it to your THR. If your 10-second pulse exceeds your THR, it is a signal to slow down your rove. If it falls short, it is a signal to speed up a little.

TABLE 4.1 TARGET HEART RATE VERSUS AGE

Your Age	Target Heart Rate (THR)
15–24	22
25–34	21
35–44	20
45–54	19
55–64	18
65–74	17
75–84	16

Learning to take your heart rate and check it against your THR is the best means possible for you to regulate your pace. On a hot day, when you should go slower, your heart rate will tell you by beating faster than normal at normal speeds. At high altitudes, when you should go slower, your heart rate will tell you again. In every condition, your heart rate is your best gauge for controlling pace.

The Concept of Distance

In roving, whether you are a walker, a full-fledged runner, or somewhere in between, the concept of distance is paramount. The objective in roving is to travel between point A and point B.

Although time is not the important factor in roving, time helps you select your distance. How far should you rove? That is, how far apart should point A and point B be? Ultimately, you should rove a distance that takes about an hour to cover. In the beginning you may not be able to stay on your feet that long. Perhaps 15 minutes is your best effort. That's fine. Rove for 15 minutes. Eventually you will be able to work up to an hour's rove with comfort.

Remember, time is only a device for helping you get some idea of how far to rove. Once you know how far you should be going, you should think of your roves as covering that distance, and remove thoughts of time from your mind.

Some writers on recreational running recommend that you set out to run a fixed amount of time each day, say 45 minutes, and ignore where or how far you run. Although it sounds a lot like roving, it is not the same. There is a small but important difference. Running (or walking) until your watch says a certain amount of time has passed can be psychologically discouraging. Time can drag as you keep looking to see if the time is up. It's like watching a pot boil. But set out to rove to the store and back and things are very different. Even if the total time is identical, the trip to the store and back will seem faster and more fun. Try it both ways and see for yourself.

How Often to Rove

Numerous studies have shown that your payoff, as far as physiological conditioning is concerned, is optimal if you rove 3 or 4 times a week. But experience with roving has shown that long-term enjoyment is greatest if you rove 6 times a week, making every other day a short, easy-paced rove.

Thus, alternate a long rove with a short, easy one. If your long rove covers 4 miles, make your short rove the next day cover only half this distance, at an easy pace.

Stretching Exercises

Running, especially on smooth surfaces like sidewalks, streets, or running tracks, builds up some muscles to a greater degree than others. This imbalance in muscle strength leads to "tightness." It gives you legs that are great for running but not very flexible for other pursuits.

Stretching exercises help overcome this imbalance by stretching the overdeveloped muscles and maintaining flexibility. Stretching is important, too, for preventing the injuries to muscles and tendons that sometimes trouble runners.

Therefore, take ten minutes before each rove to stretch the parts of your body that need stretching and to strengthen other muscle groups to balance your stronger running muscles. There are six simple exercises that can be done before any rove. These are Dr. George Sheehan's Magic Six Exercises.

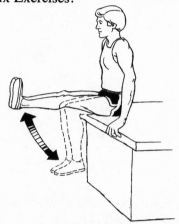

1. *Leg Raisers.* Sit on the edge of a table that is high enough to keep your feet off the floor. While sitting with your feet dangling, lift your legs gently so that they are straight out in front of you. Then return your feet to the dangle position. Repeat this lifting and lowering action for 2 minutes.

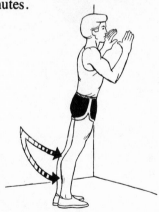

2. *Wall Push-ups.* Stand 3 feet from a wall. Now, keeping your heels on the ground, do wall push-ups. Repetition is not critical here. You are stretching your calves and the back of your knees. You can lean close to the wall and hold this position for a period of time. You may also do this exercise with one foot forward. Do this exercise for 2 minutes.

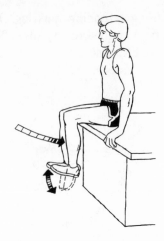

3. *Shin Strengthener*. Sit on the edge of a table and rotate your feet up and down about the ankle. Do this for 1 minute.

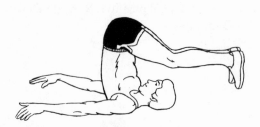

4. *Backover*. Lying on your back with your hands palms down on the floor at your hips, bring your legs as far over your head as you can. Hold for 20 seconds.

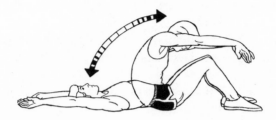

5. *Bent-leg Sit-Up.* For your stomach muscles, do bent-leg sit-ups. Do them slowly and easily for 2 minutes.

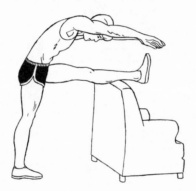

6. *Hamstring Stretches.* Place one leg on the back of a chair or other support, at an elevation suited to your height. With your other foot flat on the floor, knee locked, bend over as far as you can on your elevated leg. Hold for 30 seconds. Switch legs. Hold for 30 seconds.

Some of these exercises may be hard for you to do. Do them as best as you can. If there is one you can't do at all, don't worry about it. Perhaps you can figure out some other exercise you can do that will give you the same benefit.

In stretching, be gentle. Don't force yourself. Hard, jerky, repetitious exercises are to be avoided. Exercises that assume a position of mild stretching and hold that position for a time are preferred.

Your Exercise Prescription

The previous section contained a complete exercise prescription for you. If you follow this prescription, you will be able safely and successfully to begin a running program that will carry you to high levels of conditioning. Here is a summary of your prescription:

1. Over a period of weeks begin with walking, work up to a scout pace (alternating walking and slow jogging), and finally to continual jogging.
2. Rove 6 times a week on a long-short basis. Rove a long distance one day and a short distance at an easy pace the next.
3. Work your long roves up to a distance that will take you an hour (or more) to complete.
4. Check your heart rate in the middle and at the end of each long rove. Keep your heart rate at about your THR (see table 4.1 on page 45).
5. Warm up before each rove. Stretch, and start your rove slowly.
6. Warm down at the end of each rove. Spend 5 or 10 minutes roving at a very easy pace at the end of each rove. Warming down is essential. Coming to a quick standstill at the end of a hard rove can cause a pooling of blood in your legs and result in fainting.

Other Forms of Activity

Roving isn't the only form of activity you can select. It's just the best. It's the best physiologically because the human form is so ideally suited to it. And it is the best practically speaking because one can always do it. No special equipment other than a good pair of shoes is needed. And it can be done anywhere, at any time of year.

Some people prefer other activities. And as Dr. Jack Wilmore at the University of Arizona says: "Exercise is a lifetime pursuit. Therefore, attractive activities must be made available." So if, for example, you are an avid tennis fan and you prefer tennis above all other activities, then by all means use tennis as your form of Live Longer Now activity.

Regardless of your preferences, if you are in poor condition, 3 to 6 months of roving is essential before you begin an alternative activity. And an alternative activity has to have the potential for keeping your heart rate at your elevated THR level for a long period of time, the way roving does. The problem with some activities, and tennis is one of them, is that your heart rate may rise to a high level, too high perhaps, for a short time and then fall to a level below your THR. The time spent wandering after loose balls or conversing with friends doesn't really count as Live Longer Now activity. And time spent running like hell for a few minutes during a hard rally can be dangerous.

Competitive sports have this potential for causing unduly high heart rates. Handball, basketball, squash, and wrestling are examples of sports with this potential. So, competitive situations should be handled with a certain amount of caution.

Activities that can be treated very much like roving are swimming, rowing, bicycling, stationary bicycling, and jogging in place. They can be noncompetitive in nature, and they lend themselves to the concept of "long distance."

Activities that have no place in your exercise program, except perhaps for their amusement value, are strength exercises like weight lifting and isometrics, and pseudo exercises like bowling and golf-cart golfing.

CHAPTER 5

The World of Longevity Foods

If you look around your supermarket you will see a large assortment of foods. Your problem is to learn how to distinguish those foods that belong to the world of longevity foods and those that do not. Since you have never received any training on how to do this, you've got some learning to do.

In this chapter you'll be going back to school. You'll be learning new skills and getting homework assignments. You will learn what foods are composed of, and you will learn how this food composition should guide you when you go grocery shopping or when you go out to eat.

I urge you to read this chapter carefully. Here is where you will pick up the fundamental skills needed to make your Live Longer Now Quick Weight-Loss program work for you. When you have mastered this chapter, you will be a "world expert" in longevity eating.

Some Basic Principles

What is longevity eating? In simplest terms it is eating foods that don't contain excessive amounts of these gremlins: fat, cholesterol, salt, and sugar. Learning longevity eating is learning how to tell the difference between foods that have too many of these gremlins and foods that do not.

Let's begin the learning process with an overall look at longevity foods and other foods. This will give you a general idea of what differences there are between them. Then we'll add more detail in order to increase your discrimination.

With a few exceptions, foods as grown are a part of longevity eating. Thus corn, peas, beans, grains, tomatoes, cucumbers, rice, broccoli, barley, carrots, and potatoes are excellent longevity foods. Fruits of all kinds (in limited amounts because of the fruit sugar content) are also longevity foods. Thus, practically the entire plant kingdom is at your disposal. Table 5.1 lists many of these acceptable foods. It is a long list, and because it is so long, it shows how important the plant kingdom is in your diet.

What about the animal kingdom? Most vegetables can be eaten in unlimited quantities in longevity eating, but the same is not true when we come to animal products. Because all animal products contain cholesterol, and because many animal products are high in fat, you must limit the animal products you eat in important ways.

First, you need to limit your total meat intake to ¼ pound per day *or less*. (Lesser amounts won't harm you. I eat only an ounce of meat a day, and we serve only an ounce a day at the Institute of Health.) By meat, I mean fish, fowl, and red meat. The total of all these taken together must be kept to less than ¼ pound per day. Keeping within this limit helps control both your fat and your cholesterol intake.

Second, you must avoid certain high-cholesterol foods altogether. These foods are egg yolks, shrimp, skin, and organ meats (liver, heart, brain, etc.). Egg whites are fine, and in fact there is a delicious omelette recipe, using only egg whites, given on page 159.

Third, you must avoid certain high-fat animal products altogether. Among these are duck, goose, most lamb cuts, and all milk products except those made from skim milk.

Broadly speaking, then, longevity foods are made up of the plant kingdom and a restricted portion of the animal kingdom. Of course, even an acceptable food can be rendered unacceptable by the addition of problem ingredients during commercial processing. Thus, whereas grains ground to make whole wheat flours, breads, and cereals are fine, the addition of sugars, salts, and fats to the product will render it unacceptable. And tuna may be acceptable, but tuna canned in oil is unacceptable. Part of longevity eating, therefore, involves distinguishing between commercial products that have been spoiled by added gremlins and those that have not. I discuss this matter in greater detail in subsequent paragraphs.

Now that you have a general idea of foods to use and foods to avoid, let's add to your powers of discrimination by going through

TABLE 5.1. LONGEVITY FOODS FROM THE PLANT KINGDOM

Apples
Apple juice
Apple sauce
Apricots
Asparagus

Bananas
Barley (pearled)
Beans (white, red, pinto,
  calico, red Mexican,
  black, brown, Bayo,
  lima
Bean sprouts
Beets
Blackberries
Blueberries
Broccoli
Brussels sprouts

Cabbage (red or green)
Cantaloupe
Carrots
Cauliflower
Celery
Chard
Cherries
Chickpeas or garbanzos
Collards
Corn
Cow peas
Cranberries
Cucumbers
Currants

Eggplant
Endive or escarole

Grapefruit
Grapefruit juice
Grapefruit-orange juice
Grapes
Grape juice
Guavas

Honeydew melon

Kale
Kohlrabi

Lemons
Lemon juice
Lentils

Lettuce
Limes
Loganberries

Mangoes
Mushrooms
Muskmelons
Mustard greens

Nectarines

Oats or rolled oats or steel-
  cut oats
Okra
Onions
Oranges

Papayas
Parsley
Parsnips
Peaches
Peas
Peppers (green or red bell)
Persimmons
Pimentos
Pineapple
Pineapple juice
Plums
Potatoes
Prunes
Prune juice
Pumpkin

Radishes
Raisins
Raspberries
Rhubarb
Rice (brown, wild)
Rutabagas

Spinach
Squash (all varieties)
Strawberries
Sweet potatoes

Tangerines
Tomatoes
Tomato juice
Turnips
Turnip greens

Watermelon

the major food groups and identifying specific foods to use and specific foods to avoid.

MEATS

Use: Lean beef, pork, veal, turkey, chicken, fish, clams, lobster. Trim all visible fat before cooking. Note that fish and fowl are considered meat. Limit total meat intake to ¼ pound per day.

Avoid: Lamb, mutton, duck, goose, shrimp, crab, skin, organ meats (such as liver, heart, and kidney), and fatty meats (such as spareribs, hotdogs, sausages, fatty hamburger, bacon, and luncheon meats).

VEGETABLES, FRUITS, AND NUTS

Use: All vegetables, fruits, and juices. Limit fruits to 3 or 4 pieces a day, and limit fruit juices to 4 ounces a day.

Avoid: Nuts, avocadoes and olives (high fat contents). Also avoid packaged or canned vegetables, fruits, or juices containing sugar or salt.

BREADS, CEREALS, PASTAS, AND GRAINS

Use: Any bread made without sugar, shortening, or other sweetener or fat. (Salt in bread is often minimal. Use your taste buds as a guide. If it tastes salty, don't use it.) Unbleached whole wheat or whole grain flour preferred. Any hot cereal made without sugar, shortening, or other sweetener or fat, such as Roman Meal, Wheatena, Regular Cream of Wheat, Rolled Oats, or 4 Grain Cereal, or whole grains or whole grain mixes are preferred. Any cold cereal made without sugar, shortening, or other sweeteners or fat, such as shredded wheat (most other cold cereals are health disasters). Any whole grain pasta: spaghetti, macaroni, noodles (*not* egg noodles). Any whole grain, such as barley, corn, or rice (brown rice preferred).

Avoid: All breads or cereals made with shortening, oils, sugar, or other sweeteners. All commercial mixes containing any of these gremlins or containing whole egg or whole milk. All white-flour pastas or pastas made with whole egg.

DAIRY PRODUCTS

Use: Skim milk, nonfat milk, cheeses made from 100% skim milk (like Safeway's dry-curd cottage cheese), yogurt made from 100% skim milk, buttermilk with fat content labeled 1% or less, egg whites, or any of the cheese recipes beginning on page 166.

Avoid: Whole milk, 2% milk, low-fat milk, ordinary buttermilk, ordinary yogurt, ordinary cheeses, cheeses made from "part skim milk," and egg yolks.

FATS, OILS, BUTTERS, AND MARGARINES

Use: None of them.

Avoid: All of them, including margarines of all kinds (safflower margarines, unsaturated margarines, polyunsaturated margarines, and so on), butter, cooking oil, salad oil, olive oil, meat fat, meat drippings, lard and shortening.

DESSERTS, SNACKS, BEVERAGES, AND CONDIMENTS

Use: Fruit; crackers made without sugar, shortening, and so forth; acceptable breads; decaffeinated beverages; linden flower tea (one of the few harmless teas); spices of all kinds (not premixed spices, which are usually salty); any of the desserts beginning on page 215.

Avoid: All pies, cakes, pastries, and so on, and baking items containing shortening. All fried foods like potato chips and french fries. All sugared drinks and candy. All syrups and syrup-packed fruits. All ice cream, sherbets, and puddings. All forms of salt including salt substitutes.

The Composition of Foods

Longevity eating can be described by the foods you eat and those you don't eat. That is exactly how I have tried to describe it on the preceding pages. But longevity eating can be characterized in other ways as well. This section characterizes longevity eating by the composition, or makeup, of the foods eaten.

Every bite of food you eat can be broken down into these five substances:

1. Carbohydrates
2. Protein
3. Fat
4. Vitamins and minerals
5. Water, fiber, and other nonnutritive material

Your bites will differ only on how much of each substance the foods you eat contain. When you eat a bite of sugar candy, you are eating 100 percent carbohydrate, and virtually nothing else. When you eat a bite of butter, you are eating nearly 100 percent fat, and little else. When you eat a bite of whole-grain bread, you are eating a significant amount of all five substances.

Longevity eating is striking in the matter of where the calories come from. (We get calories only from the carbohydrates, fat, and protein we eat. There are no calories associated with vitamins, minerals, water, fiber, or other nonnutritive substances.) Longevity eating is unusual in that a large part of the calories in longevity food come from carbohydrates. Protein and fat from a much smaller percentage of the calories. Specifically, 78 percent or more of the calories come from carbohydrate, about 10 percent come from fat, and about 12 percent come from protein. Compare these percentages with the diet of the average American. The average American takes in only 46 percent of his or her calories as carbohydrates but takes in a whopping 42 percent of calories as fat. Protein intake is about the same in both diets—12 percent.

High carbohydrate intake is a key feature of longevity eating. Furthermore, the carbohydrates in longevity eating are exclusively *complex* carbohydrates: foods as grown. Complex carbohydrates are the trademark of the plant world. All plants contain complex carbohydrates, which are used for supportive structures in the plant and, in the form of starches, for energy storage. These complex carbohydrates are ideal sources of energy for the human body, burning with 100 percent efficiency and leaving no by-products other than carbon dioxide and water.

A distinction must be drawn between complex carbohydrates, which are a part of longevity eating, and simple carbohydrates, which are not. Simple carbohydrates are nothing more than predigested complex carbohydrates. Sugar, honey, syrup, molasses, and foods made from them are examples of simple carbohydrates. By breaking down complex carbohydrates into their simplest parts, by digestion or by commercial processing, simple carbohydrates are produced.

Simple carbohydrates have a number of distinct disadvantages. They are without plant fiber, they are generally devoid of vitamins and minerals, and they are caloric dynamite. Moreover, their reaction in the body is physiologically harmful: Blood sugar levels and blood insulin levels are both substantially increased, at the expense of increased blood fats, increased fat storage, and probable damage to the body's appetite-control mechanisms.

Primitive people in general fall into the class of people around the world who engage in longevity eating naturally. Under primitive conditions, longevity foods are the only foods available. They are the foods that humankind has evolved with over the last several million years.

The Tarahumara Indians of northern Mexico, cut off from the influence of modern civilization by the rugged Sierra Madre, use longevity foods exclusively. The Tarahumara diet is 75 percent complex carbohydrates, 12 percent fat, and 13 percent protein. It consists mostly of vegetables, beans, corn, and the like, supplemented by a small amount of meat (a few ounces a week). Heart disease, high blood pressure, and atherosclerosis are unknown among the Tarahumara, as is overweight.

Bite for bite, longevity food has less than half the calories of the food eaten by the average American. Bite for bite, longevity food has over three times the fiber of the average American's food.

Longevity eating excludes foods that have long been viewed as vitamin-rich—liver, for example. Nevertheless, because longevity eating includes a rich variety of grains, vegetables, fruits, and animal products, an ample supply of vitamins and minerals results. Table 5.2 analyzes the nutritional composition of a day's meals mimicking those served at the Institute of Health. Even though the calorie intake is less than 2000 calories, vitamin and mineral intakes meet or exceed the daily allowances recommended by the Food and Nutrition Board of the National Academy of Sciences.

When we discuss recommended daily allowances, we put our finger on another important aspect of longevity eating: Longevity eating seeks to control *excesses* in the food we eat. This is different from the ideas of classical nutrition that seek to control *deficiencies* in the food we eat. Thus the Food and Nutrition Board is concerned that we don't get too little in the way of iron, say, or of vitamin C. Longevity eating is concerned that we don't get too much in the way of fat, cholesterol, or the like. Both views are critically important to health.

Identifying Longevity Foods by Food Composition

The previous sections should have taught you that longevity foods can be characterized by how much fat, complex carbohydrate, and protein content they have. Now let's have some fun and look at 100 common foods and discuss their fat, complex carbohydrate, and protein contents. Knowing these contents, you should be able to tell which foods to accept and which to reject. Here are some rules of thumb:

1. Since this list contains mostly unprocessed foods, you don't have to worry about simple versus complex carbohydrates. You may assume that all carbohydrates are complex. That's good. No food in this list needs to be rejected because it has sugar, honey, or other noncomplex carbohydrates in it. None does.

2. Any food, except meat, that contains more than 10 percent fat, should be rejected. Meat (meaning red meat, fish, and fowl) adds both undesirable fat and cholesterol. But our limitation of

TABLE 5.2. NUTRITIONAL COMPOSITION OF MEALS MIMICKING THOSE OF THE INSTITUTE OF HEALTH

	Calories	Protein in Calories	Fat in Calories	Carbohydrates in Calories	Calcium mg	Phosphorous mg	Iron mg	Sodium mg	Potassium mg	Vitamin A Int units	Thiamin mg	Riboflavin mg	Niacin mg	Ascorbic Acid mg
Breakfast: Cereal	404	61	17	335	183	484	4	61	728	123	.53	.36	5	8
Toast	97	14	5	82	13	113	1.1	.6	105	—	14	.04	1	—
Orange	81	5	3	73	68	33	.65	2	331	330	.17	.01	.65	83
Lunch: Salad	150	19	7.2	117	157	165	3.8	326	1369	2765	.35	2.8	2.7	92
Bread	97	14	5	82	13	113	1.1	.6	105	—	14	.04	1.3	—
Pea Soup	118	25	3.4	84	67	143	2.3	143	457	663	.35	.18	3.2	44
Dinner: Bread	194	28	10	164	26	226	2.2	1.2	210	—	28	.08	2.6	—
Corn	96	9	8.4	82	3	111	.7	—	280	400	.15	.12	1.7	12
Soup	86	12	4.4	71	65	90	5.6	25	883	3527	.19	.13	2.3	81
Main Course	538	79	34	427	281	568	96	560	2477	4615	29	3.2	8.4	156
Dessert	61	.67	5.2	55	7	11	.33	1	115	95	2.8	2.7	.08	4
Total (rounded)	1922	267	103	1572	883	2057	118	1120	7060	12,518	90	10	29	480
% of total		14%	5%	82%										

no more than ¼ pound of meat per day keeps both these elements in check.

3. Regardless of its fat content, a high-cholesterol food must be rejected (organ meats, skin, egg yolk, and certain shellfish).

Below is a list of fruits and fruit juices. Look it over, then let's discuss it in the paragraph that follows the list.

	Protein (%)	Fat (%)	Carbohydrate (%)
Apples	1	9	90
Apple juice	1	0	99
Apple sauce (unsweetened)	2	4	95
Apricots	7	3	89
Apricots canned in water	6	2	91
Avocados	5	84	11
Bananas	4	2	94
Blueberries	4	7	89
Cantaloupe	8	3	90
Cherries (sweet)	6	4	90
Coconut	3	85	10
Grapefruit	4	2	94
Nectarines	3	0	96
Oranges	9	3	89
Orange juice	12	2	86
Peaches	5	2	92
Pineapple	3	3	95
Strawberries	6	11	82
Tangerines	6	4	90
Tomatoes	18	8	74
Watermelon	7	7	86

Several things are obvious from the list. First, except for tomatoes, all the fruits are low in protein. Second, except for coconuts and avocados, all the fruits are high in complex carbohydrates. Third, only the coconuts and avocados are high in fat, and they are very high. Thus, from this list we may conclude that *coconut and avocados should be excluded from longevity eating,* but all the other fruits are O.K.

The list that follows shows grain and flour (unbleached whole wheat flour). These excellent longevity foods are uniformly low in fat and high in complex carbohydrates. Other grains such as corn, wild rice, and buckwheat are also excellent.

	Protein (%)	Fat (%)	Carbohydrate (%)
Barley (pearl)	8	2	90
Rice (brown)	7	4	89
Wheat	16	6	78
Flour (whole wheat)	16	6	78

Take a look at the legumes (beans and peas) in the list below. Except for soybeans, they are all remarkably low in fat, high in complex carbohydrates, and surprisingly high in protein. Soybeans must be excluded from longevity eating because of their high fat content. So, enjoy these beans, peas, and lentils—but stay away from soybeans.

	Protein (%)	Fat (%)	Carbohydrate (%)
Red beans	23	4	73
Pinto beans	23	3	74
Lima beans	20	4	76
Green beans	24	6	70
Chick-peas (garbanzos)	20	11	70
Lentils	25	3	71
Soybeans	34	39	28

Nuts are an eye-opener. Below are listed peanuts, cashews, and water chestnuts. Peanuts and cashews are typical of all nuts except chestnuts and water chestnuts. Nuts have a fat content of 70 to 80 percent and are therefore unacceptable as longevity foods. Chestnuts and water chestnuts are the only acceptable nuts.

	Protein (%)	Fat (%)	Carbohydrate (%)
Peanuts	16	70	14
Cashews	12	73	15
Water chestnuts	6	2	92

Before leaving the question of nuts, let's face up to a question you may already have formed: Nuts are seemingly so natural a food, why would they be harmful to man? The answer may be that nuts, while available in small quantities to evolutionary man, probably did not form a significant part of his daily diet. In spite of the high fat content of nuts, it is doubtful whether evolutionary man was able to find and eat enough nuts to raise his daily fat intake much. For modern man, aided by modern cultivation and food processing, this is a different story. Modern man can take in *any amount* of nuts per day—hands full, bags full, or pounds of nuts—and can increase his fat intake to any level he desires in this way. So, while nuts have been around a long time, and in very small quantities may cause no harm, in the quantities we are now able to obtain, they are definitely harmful.

The list that follows is for meat (red meats, fish, and fowl). It won't take you long to realize how high in fat meat can be. Regular hamburger is over 70 percent fat, and even lean hamburger is over 50 percent fat. This is why I urge you to eat only the *leanest* cuts of meat and only in quantities *less than* ¼ pound per day. In selecting longevity meats, select only those whose fat contents are under 40 percent.

	Protein (%)	Fat (%)	Carbohydrate (%)
Barracuda	78	22	0
Beef			
T-bone (good grade, separable lean)	63	37	0
hamburger (extra lean)	63	37	0
hamburger (lean)	45	55	0
hamburger (regular)	28	72	0
Chicken			
breast	79	21	0
drumstick	69	31	0
Duck meat	21	79	0
Halibut	88	12	0
Lamb leg (choice)	64	36	0
Lobster	78	20	2

	Protein (%)	Fat (%)	Carbohydrate (%)
Salmon			
red Sockeye	50	50	0
pink	61	39	0
Scallops	79	5	16
Swordfish	68	22	0
Tuna (canned in water)	94	6	0
Turkey (light meat)	89	11	0
young bird, light meat	95	5	0
Veal			
chunk (thin class)	60	40	0
loin (thin class)	53	47	0

The next list is for dairy products. Cheeses like Cheddar, blue, Roquefort, Camembert, Swiss, and Parmesan are uniformly high in fat (60 to 75 percent fat). Cottage cheese is also alarmingly high in fat (36 percent) unless it is dry-curd (also called uncreamed) cottage cheese. Even though 36 percent isn't as high as a few of the allowable meats, since there is no built-in control on cottage cheese (similar to the ¼ pound per day limit on meat), only uncreamed (dry-curd) cottage cheese should be used. Obviously egg yolks are out and egg whites are in. Whey, the liquid left over from cheese making, is an acceptable longevity food. And only skim milk should be used.

	Protein (%)	Fat (%)	Carbohydrate (%)
Cheeses			
Cheddar	27	72	2
cottage (creamed)	54	36	10
cottage (uncreamed)	83	3	13
Eggs			
yolks	19	79	1
whites	93	0	7
Milk, skim	42	2	55
Whey	14	10	76

The next list is for vegetables. Need we say anything? All vegetables are excellent longevity foods. Complex carbohydrates are uniformly high and fats are uniformly low. Use them with variety in unlimited quantities.

	Protein (%)	Fat (%)	Carbohydrate (%)
Asparagus	26	8	66
Beets	11	2	87
Bell peppers	24	9	67
Broccoli	33	9	58
Brussels sprouts	30	9	61
Cabbage	15	8	77
Carrots	8	5	87
Cauliflower	30	7	63
Celery	15	5	80
Corn, sweet	9	9	82
Eggplant	13	8	79
Lettuce (iceberg)	19	7	77
Mushrooms	32	11	57
Onions	11	2	87
Parsnips	7	6	87
Peas	24	5	71
Potatoes	8	1	91
Spinach	33	11	56
Squash (summer)	16	5	79

How to Read Labels

Learning to read the labels on commercial foods is your key to distinguishing longevity foods from other foods in your supermarket. Longevity foods may be identified by three characteristics:

1. Longevity foods are low in fat—less than 10% of total calories.
2. Longevity foods don't contain added sugars or salt.
3. Longevity foods don't contain artificial colors or artificial flavors.

The labels on canned and packaged foods usually contain enough information to decide whether or not these three characteristics are present. Let's talk a little more about each of the items.

Reading the Label for Fat Content

Determining fat content can be tricky. Fat content is not always given on foods, and when it is, it is often given in a form that is useless to you. For instance, whole milk is advertised as 3½ percent fat. At first glance you might think to yourself: "Aha! The fat content of this product is less than 10 percent. It must be longevity food." But you would be wrong. Milk is actually about 48 percent fat, fourteen times as high as the amount advertised.

What is the problem? Well, the manufacturer is giving you the percent of fat by weight rather than by the amount of calories the fat provides. You want to know the fat content by calorie contribution. Fat content by weight is a useless piece of information. You don't care what the percent of fat by weight is, because the weight of food is often totally unrelated to its food value. Milk, for example, is 90 percent water. Water has no food value whatsoever. All the food-value material in milk taken together only accounts for 10 percent of the weight of the milk. It's no wonder that fat, one of the elements with food value, only comes up to 4 percent of the total weight, even though it comes to almost 50 percent of the total calories.

With milk and milk products, the easiest way around this problem is simply to reject any product not made from 100 percent skim milk. This means that low-fat milk, 2 percent milk, low-fat yogurt, and low-fat cottage cheese are out. However, 1 percent buttermilk is in.

Many products today carry "nutrition information" on the label. And often this nutrition information will give you the information you need in order to know fat content (by calories, not by weight). Usually nutrition information will give you these two bits of information: (1) total calories in one serving and (2) grams of fat in one serving. You'll have to do a little arithmetic, but this information is all you need.

Here's what you do. Multiply the number of grams of fat they give you by 100. You can do that in your head. It's easy to multiply by 100. Now compare this with the total number of calories in the serving. Is it less than or equal to the total number of calories in a serving? Yes or no.

If yes, you've got a longevity food. If no, you don't. With practice you can get so proficient that you can tell a longevity food (as far as fat content is concerned) by a mere glance at the label.

Example 1: Zinger's Homemade Bread
Serving size, 1 slice
Calories per serving, 30
Grams of carbohydrates, 5.9
Grams of protein, 1.0
Grams of fat, .3

In the above example there are only two things of interest: calories per serving, 30; and grams of fat, .3. Multiplying .3 by 100 we get 30. This is equal to the number of calories in a serving. Thus Zinger's Homemade Bread is longevity food. Had it been less than 30, it would still have been longevity food. But if it had been greater than 30, it would not have been.

Example 2: Grandma's Butter Bread
Serving size, 1 ounce
Calories per serving, 97
Grams of carbohydrates, 15.0
Grams of protein, 2.5
Grams of fat, 3.1

In Example 2, calories per serving are 97, and grams of fat are 3.1. Multiplying 3.1 by 100 we get 310. Is 310 less than or equal to 97? No. It is greater than 97. So Grandma's Butter Bread is *not* longevity food.

Sometimes there is no nutrition information on the label. If the food seems to be an acceptable food according to what you have learned in the previous pages, your task is easy. Take a look at the ingredients list. (All products have an ingredients list, whether or not there is a "nutrition information" section on the label. An ingredients list is simply a list of everything in the product, usually in the order of quantity; largest quantity comes first on the list.) Take a look at the ingredients list, and if neither fat, lard, shortening, oil, nor margarine is listed there, the product is a longevity food. But if any of these items is listed, reject the food. This is playing it safe. With sufficient nutrition information you might decide that even with some fat as an ingredient, the quantity is less than 10 percent and therefore safe. But without nutrition information, you're stuck. If a fat appears in the ingredients list, the food must be rejected out of hand.

Reading the Label for Sugar or Salt

The easiest way to find out about sugar and salt is to read the ingredients portion of the label. If salt or any of the many forms of sugar is listed, reject the item. Sugar includes sugar, raw sugar, brown sugar, corn sweetners, corn syrup, syrup, molasses, honey, and the "oses": mannose, dextrose, maltose, and the like.

Frequently the amount of salt used in commercial bread is small and of no health consequence. In fact, salt in bread is ordinarily used to control the rate at which the bread rises rather than to control flavor. For this reason, even bread with salt may be considered longevity food, provided that you use your taste buds as a guide. If the bread tastes salty in any way, reject it.

Occasionally a product will specify the percentage of salt it contains by dry weight. If it does, and if it is *less than 1 percent by dry weight,* the product may be used. Otherwise it should be rejected.

For someone on a diet of 2000 calories a day, this rule on salt usage guarantees that salt intake will be no more than 5 grams per day. The actual amount of salt taken in depends on the foods eaten, but may be in the neighborhood of 2 grams a day or even lower. The average American's intake of 15 grams daily is significantly higher than this figure.

Reading the Label for Chemical Additives

Food manufacturers may add hundreds of chemicals to foods at their whim. These chemicals are listed on the government's GRAS list (Generally Regarded As Safe list). These chemicals are added by the food processor for only one reason: to increase the profitability of his product. They are used for flavoring, coloring, texture, consistency, and so forth. In general, systematic attempts to determine the safety of chemicals on the GRAS list have been slow in coming.

Many chemicals are there almost out of habit because they have been used by food manufacturers for so many years.

When studies have been done, the results have often been shocking. Saccharin and the cyclamates, used as sweeteners, have been shown to cause cancer. Nitrites, used as preservatives in meats, have been shown to produce nitrosamines, also powerful cancer-causing agents. Even the dye used in maraschino cherries, the notorious Red 4, has been shown to cause cancer.

In spite of claims from food manufacturers that chemical additives are necessary for the production of palatable foods, it is hard to believe that there is any real potential for good from chemical additives. The potential for harm is clearly large. This is especially true when we realize how *many* chemicals are in our foods. Ultimately, some may prove safe, but others are bound to be harmful. And we get them *all*, safe and unsafe alike, unless we reject foods with artificial additives out of hand.

For all these reasons, longevity foods must be only those that have not been spoiled by the addition of artificial colorings or flavorings. Even though it is hard to draw the line between what is artificial and what is natural, and even though some "natural" products are undoubtedly harmful, the only way out of the morass of GRAS additives is to follow this rule: When you read the label, watch for artificial additives. Where they are listed, reject the food.

The Cholesterol Content of Foods

Longevity eating is characterized by a much lower intake of cholesterol than is usual in ordinary American eating. The average American eats well over 600 mg of cholesterol per day. Using longevity foods you will be eating less than 100 mg of cholesterol per day—a substantial reduction, and an excellent line of defense against heart disease and other degenerative diseases.

The way you guarantee yourself less than 100 mg of cholesterol a day is to limit your daily meat intake to less than ¼ pound and avoid all high-cholesterol products (such things as egg yolks and animal organ meats like liver and heart). To learn even more about the cholesterol content of foods and what can and cannot be eaten, look at Table 5.3, the Cholesterol Content in 3½ Ounces of Common Foods. This is an important table. You should look it over carefully, for it has a lot to teach you.

Assume that you are eating 3½ ounces of meat (just under ¼ pound) a day. To be sure that you don't get more than 100 mg of cholesterol a day, all you have to do is limit yourself to those foods in Table 5.3 that have less than 100 mg of cholesterol.

Suppose, for instance, you sliced a piece of lean beef and trimmed off the visible fat. According to the table, if you cooked that meat and ate it, your cholesterol intake would be only 65 mg for the day—well under the 100 mg allowed.* On the other hand, the table shows that if you were to cook 3½ ounces of beef liver, you would be eating 300 mg of cholesterol—far above the allotment.†

Table 5.3 can guide you as to the different kinds of meats available and whether or not they are allowable *as far as their cholesterol content is concerned.*

Here you should be careful. Just because a food has a low level of cholesterol does not mean it is a longevity food. After all, there are other factors in longevity eating besides cholesterol, among them sugar, fat, and salt. Thus cakes, pies, and candies, which have low levels of cholesterol, are excluded on the basis of their sugar contents. Cheeses and mayonnaise, which have medium levels of cholesterol, are excluded on the basis of their fat contents. And caviar is excluded on the basis of both its salt content and its cholesterol content—not to mention its cost.

A feature that becomes apparent from an inspection of Table 5.3 is the absence of vegetables, fruits, grains, or beans from the table. Cholesterol is characteristic of the animal kingdom. All animals make it, and it occurs in every animal product. Vegetables don't

---

*Don't be confused by the fact that the table shows cooked beef as having 91 mg of cholesterol while raw beef has only 65. Cholesterol content doesn't actually change during cooking. The higher figure would result only if you weighed your portion after cooking, instead of before cooking as you are supposed to. The value for cooked meat is higher than the value for raw meat because the cooked meat is more condensed, having lost moisture during the cooking process.
†Why, you might ask, does Table 5.3 show cholesterol values for 3½ ounces instead of 4 ounces? After all, 4 ounces = ¼ pound and you are *allowed* up to ¼ pound of meat a day. The reason is that 3½ ounces is equal to 100 grams, and cholesterol tables all come in 100-gram measures. And 3½ ounces is close enough to 4 ounces for our purposes.

TABLE 5.3. CHOLESTEROL CONTENT IN 3½ OUNCES
OF COMMON FOODS

Food and Description	*Cholesterol (mg)*
Beef	
Retail cuts; total edible, raw	68
Lean, trimmed of separable fat	
raw	65
cooked	(91)[a]
Beef and Vegetable Stew	
cooked (home recipe, with lean beef chunk)	26
canned	14
Chipped, Creamed, dried beef	21
Potpie	
home-prepared, baked	21
commercial, frozen, unheated	18
Brains, raw	>2000
Butter	250
Buttermilk, fluid, cultured, made from	
nonfat fluid milk	2
Chicken	
Whole	
raw	
flesh, skin, and giblets (refuse:	98
bones, 30%)	
flesh and skin only	81
cooked, flesh and skin only	87
Breast	
raw (refuse: bones, 21%)	67
cooked	
total edible	80
meat only	79
Drumstick	
raw (refuse: bone, 40%)	88
cooked	
total edible	91
meat only	91

[a] Numbers in parentheses denote imputed values.

TABLE 5.3 (continued)

Food and Description	Cholesterol (mg)
Fricassee, cooked, from home recipe	40
À la king, cooked, from home recipe	76
Potpie, home prepared, baked	31
Commercial, frozen, unheated	13
chicken and noodles, cooked, from home recipe	40
chop suey, with meat cooked from home recipe	26
canned	12
chow mein, chicken (without noodles) cooked, from home recipe	31
canned	3
Clams, raw	50
Cod	
Raw	
whole (refuse: head, tail, fins, entrails, scales, bones, and skin, 69%)	50
flesh only	50
Crab, all kinds	100
Deviled	102
Imperial	140
Eggs, chicken	
Whole	
raw or cooked with nothing added (refuse: shell, 11%)	504
frozen, commercial	515
dried, commercial	1900
Whites, fresh, frozen and dried	0
Yolks	
raw or cooked with nothing added	1480
frozen, commercial	1270
dried, commercial	2630
Flounder, raw	50
Frog legs, raw (refuse: bones, 35%)	50

TABLE 5.3 (continued)

Food and Description	Cholesterol (mg)
Gizzard	
Chicken, all classes	
raw	145
cooked	(195)
Turkey, all classes	
raw	145
cooked	229
Haddock, raw	60
Halibut, raw	50
Heart	
Beef	
raw	150
cooked	(274)
Chicken, all classes	
raw	170
cooked	(231)
Turkey, all classes	
raw	150
cooked	238
Herring	
Raw	85
Canned, plain, solids and liquid	(97)
Kidneys	
Raw	375
Cooked	(804)
Lamb, composite of retail cuts	
Total edible	
raw	71
cooked	(98)
Lean, trimmed of separable fat	
raw	70
cooked	(100)
Liver	
Beef, calf, hog, and lamb	
raw	300
cooked	(438)

TABLE 5.3 (continued)

Food and Description	Cholesterol (mg)
Chicken, all classes	
raw	555
cooked	(746)
Turkey, all classes	
raw	435
cooked	599
Lobster, cooked, meat only	85
Newburg	182
Mackerel	
Raw	95
Canned, solids and liquid	(94)
Milk	
Fresh	
Whole	14
Low-fat	
1% fat with 1% to 2% nonfat milk solids added	6
2% fat with 1% to 2% nonfat milk solids added	9
Nonfat (skim)	2
Canned, concentrated, undiluted evaporated	
unsweetened	31
condensed, sweetened	34
Dry	
whole, instant	109
nonfat, instant	22
Noodles	
Whole egg	
dry form	94
cooked	31
Chow mein, canned	12
Oysters	
Raw	50
Canned, solids and liquids	(45)

TABLE 5.3 (continued)

Food and Description	Cholesterol (mg)
Stew, home prepared	
1 part oysters to 2 parts milk by volume	26
1 part oysters to 3 parts milk by volume	24
Pork, composite of lean retail cuts	
Total edible	
raw	62
cooked	(89)
Lean, trimmed of separable fat	
raw	60
cooked	(88)
Potatoes	
Au gratin, made with milk and cheese	15
Scalloped, made with milk	6
Rabbit, domesticated, flesh only	
Raw	65
Cooked	(91)
Roe, salmon, raw	360
Salmon, sockeye or red	35
Sardines, canned in oil	
Solids and liquid	(120)
Drained solids	140
Scallops, muscle only	
Raw	35
Steamed	(53)
Shrimp	150
Spaghetti with meat balls	
Cooked, from home recipe	30
Canned	9
Sweetbreads (thymus)	
Raw	250
Cooked	(466)
Trout, raw, flesh only	55
Tuna, canned in water, solids and liquid	(63)

TABLE 5.3 (continued)

Food and Description	*Cholesterol (mg)*
Turkey, all classes	
Whole	
raw	
flesh, skin, and giblets (refuse: bone, 27%)	82
flesh and skin only	74
cooked	
flesh, skin, and giblets	105
flesh and skin only	93
Light meat without skin	
raw	60
cooked	77
Dark meat without skin	
raw	75
cooked	101
Skin	
raw	110
cooked	127
Potpie	
home prepared, baked	31
commercial, frozen, unheated	9
Veal, composite of retail cuts	71

contain cholesterol. The cholesterol content of the average vegetable is a solid zero.

It is easy to confuse cholesterol with fat, so let's make it clear right now: They are different. We need to control both cholesterol and fat, and they are controlled in different ways. Cholesterol occurs only in animal products and is controlled by limiting meat to less than ¼ pound a day and avoiding high-cholesterol products. Fat occurs in both animal and vegetable products (nuts, avocados, olives, vegetable oils, for example) and is controlled by avoiding fatty animal products like cheeses, bacon, and sausage altogether, as well as avoiding fatty and oily vegetable products.

Homework

Here are some homework assignments that will help sharpen your ability to discriminate longevity foods from other foods.

A. Go to your supermarket and select two shopping carts. Select commercially packaged or canned foods at random from your supermarket shelves. For each food selected, read the label and decide whether or not it is a longevity food. If it is a longevity food, drop it in one basket. If it is not, drop it in the other basket. In this way you will have a random sample of supermarket longevity and nonlongevity foods in two baskets. Which basket fills up fastest? Are you proficient at making determinations of fat content by mental arithmetic? Can you distinguish fats and sugar in an ingredients list?

B. Go to your cupboard and read the labels on your canned and packaged foods. What percentage of your foods would you say are longevity foods? Did you spot the sugar and salt in canned vegetables? Did you notice the many packaged foods with added oils and fats? Did you remember the salty things like cocktail onions, pickles, and salt-cured meats? How about the mayonnaise, imitation mayonnaise, relish, ketchup, and soy sauce? All have salt, sugar, or high fat contents.

C. Problems (For answers, see page 219.)

The two ingredients lists below are from popular, commercially packaged foods available in your supermarket. See if you can identify unacceptable ingredients in each list.

1. Zowie Cereal
   Ingredients: sugar, corn flour, oat flour, wheat flour, salt, coconut oil, artificial flavor, natural flavor, BHT, vitamins and minerals

2. Mod Muffin Mix
   Ingredients: bleached white flour, sugar, vegetable shortening, nonfat dry milk, dried egg yolk, leavening, salt, artificial flavor, artificial color

From the two nutrition information labels following, see if you can determine whether either or both of these products is less than 10% fat by calorie contribution.

3. Buttermilk Biscuit Mix Nutrition Information:
   Serving size, ½ cup
   Calories per serving, 240
   Grams of carbohydrate, 38
   Grams of protein, 4
   Grams of fat, 8
4. French Rolls Nutrition Information:
   Serving size, 1 roll
   Calories per serving, 100
   Grams of carbohydrate, 3
   Grams of protein, 18
   Grams of fat, 1

Meal Planning

Although we will be talking about meal planning in this section, our only interest at this point is to show you how to plan longevity meals with enough variety to satisfy your needs. We're not interested in amounts. In fact, we want to explore ways to get plenty of delicious longevity foods before you, in a manner most convenient to you. Later on, in Chapters 8 and 9, we'll come back to the question of amounts and show you how to gain precision control over the amount of food you eat.

Meal planning can be quite complex. You can go into detailed menus covering days or even weeks. In fact, we'll talk about just such detailed menus in the paragraphs below, because it's an educational experience to see what detailed meal planning is like, even if you never do it.

Meal planning can also be simple. After all, food is basically simple. Corn, peas, rice, bread, vegetables, fruits, fish, tomatoes, lettuce, and grains are the foods humans thrive on. You can't go wrong planning for, and fixing, these foods. They are always available at your supermarket, and almost any means by which you render them edible will produce acceptable foods and effective meals.

Think about it. People have been eating these foods for millions of years. They have boiled them, baked them, broiled them, and eaten them raw. They have savored them all ways.

Many of us have gotten so used to packaged convenience foods and junk food that we have forgotten that *all* these slickly packaged items started out as natural foods like grains and vegetables. Processing may have obliterated even the memory of the natural foods a convenience food was made from, but these natural foods are there nevertheless. So, in meal planning remember: It is the simplest thing in the world to pick out a variety of natural foods to eat. They are always available at your supermarket; they are the easiest foods to prepare; they are ultimately healthful; and their delicate flavors have been pleasing human tastes since the beginning of time.

The Easy Way

Because I am busy and don't have a lot of time to spend thinking about food, I like to plan meals the easy way. Easy planning relies on two things: (1) a certain amount of routine, and (2) the use of dishes that are easy to make.

What constitutes an easy dish depends on you. What is easy for you might be hard for me. Likewise, an eating routine that works well for me might not work well for you. To show you the routine I use, and the dishes I make, a typical week's menu for me is shown below.

Breakfast
    Cooked cereal (Cracked wheat, rolled oats, or 4-grain cereal.
        Instant cooked cereals are never used.)
    Banana slices on cereal, topped with cinnamon and skim milk
    Toast (bread recipe on page 212)
    6 ounces grapefruit juice or half grapefruit

Lunch
    Some of last night's leftover dinner
    Bread
    Lettuce, tomatoes, vegetable salad (also from last night?)

Dinner
    One or two of these entrées:
        Mixed bean dish
        Corn and/or rice

Fish fillet

Spaghetti (whole wheat) and spaghetti sauce

Steamed or pressure cooked vegetables

Boiled, baked, or scalloped potatoes

Macaroni and white sauce

A tossed lettuce, tomato, and vegetable salad

A serving of bread (no butter allowed or needed on delicious longevity bread)

A beverage: water, linden tea, or 6 ounces skim milk

This menu is routine for several reasons. First, breakfast is the same every morning. The only variation is in the cereal used. Believe it or not, this hearty breakfast is not only delicious, but I never tire of it. The small change from one hot cereal to another provides all the variety needed for me—and for most people who have adopted it. It is the standard breakfast at the Institute of Health. For a little more variety in breakfast see the breakfast dishes beginning on page 159 or the Breakfast chapter of the *Live Longer Now Cookbook.*

Second, the menu uses staple items that you always have on hand: bread, beans, macaroni, spaghetti, corn, rice, and potatoes.

Third, lunch is *always* some of last night's dinner. It is an interesting feature of longevity foods that leftovers work out well. Because of the low fat and low salt content, these foods usually taste as good the next day as they do the day they are made. And because the fat content is low, leftovers can be eaten cold or hot, a feature ordinary food does not always have.

Nothing could be simpler than the entrées I eat for dinner. None of them requires a recipe. Once you've learned to make spaghetti or beans or macaroni or steamed vegetables or baked fish fillet or boiled corn on the cob or rice, you can whip up an entrée without a recipe, and use seasonings or chopped vegetables as flavor enhancers as you see fit. If you've ever done any cooking you'll know what I mean. If you haven't, the *Live Longer Now Cookbook* will get you started.

The Comprehensive Way to Plan Meals

My wife tells me that most people are not satisfied with the simple meals I eat. She says people want more variety, more taste experiences, and a higher palatation from food they eat. She is probably right.

One way to get more variety and palatation is to plan a more comprehensive menu with more sophisticated dishes. I call this the "hard way to do meal planning," but I'm not completely serious when I say this. To many of you this may be the only acceptable way to plan meals, and it's not really "hard."

A comprehensive meal plan begins with a comprehensive menu. Table 5.4 is an example of menus for a week. Six days of meals are shown. The seventh day, Saturday, is set aside to finish up leftovers and make plans for next week's meals. This particular menu happens to be the first six days' meals served in the Institute of Health's 10-day residential treatment program for overweight. We have found that these meals are well accepted and form a good introduction to longevity eating. The menu begins with pancakes and berry sauce for breakfast Sunday morning, and ends with an all-time favorite: pizza with ice-cream-pie dessert on Friday night. It has my favorite dinner, **Arroz con Pollo** (rice with chicken), on Wednesday and my favorite dessert, **Apple Bake,** on Thursday.*

The meal plan dictates your grocery list. A complete grocery list, computed as if you were shopping for a family of four, has been made up for the menus and is shown in Table 5.5. This list shows you all the things you need to buy: spices, baking ingredients, canned goods, milk, meat, and produce. It even breaks down the perishables—milk, meat, and produce—into two groups: those you would buy on Saturday for use on Monday through Wednesday, and those you would buy on Wednesday for use on Thursday through Saturday. Of course, some things on the list would already be in your cupboards. Spices, canned goods, and vinegar are examples of items you might already have on hand.

---

*Recipes for dishes in **boldface** type appear in this book, beginning on page 157. You can look them up easily in the Recipe Title Index.

TABLE 5.4. ONE WEEK'S SAMPLE MENUS

SUNDAY	MONDAY
Breakfast	*Breakfast*
Velvety Pancakes	Hot cereal (e.g., **Steel-Cut**
Strawberry Sauce	**Oatmeal)**
Blueberry Sauce	Orange slices
Grapefruit	Toast
Lunch	*Lunch*
Salad	**Cream of Pea Soup**
Creamy Salad Dressing	Salad
Crackers	Salad dressing (**Garlic and**
Greek Lentil Soup	**Vinegar Dressing)**
Dinner	*Dinner*
Salad	Salad
Chicken Laced Manicotti	**Enchiladas**
Chicken Stuffing	**Quick Tortilla Chips**
Mushroom Sauce	**Chili Salsa**
Fresh steamed cauliflower	**Spanish Brown Rice**
and broccoli	
	Dessert
Dessert	Piece of fruit
Fruit salad	

TABLE 5.4 (continued)

TUESDAY	WEDNESDAY
Breakfast	*Breakfast*
Hot cereal (e.g., 7-grain cereal with banana slices, cinnamon & skimmed milk) **Breakfast Bagels** ½ Grapefruit	Hot cereal with bananas Toast ¼ Cantaloupe
Lunch	*Lunch*
Salad **Potato Soup** Crackers (e.g., Finn Crisps)	**Minestrone with Rice** Salad Salad Dressing (**Tangy Salad Dressing**)
Dinner	*Dinner*
Salad **Nada's Beef Cabbage Rolls** **Stove Potatoes** Steamed zucchini Bread	**Crock Pot Soup** **Arroz Con Pollo** Vegetable of your choice Bread Salad
Dessert	*Dessert*
Piece of fruit	Fruit salad **Lucinda's Grain Dessert**

TABLE 5.4 (continued)

THURSDAY

Breakfast

Hot cereal with bananas and
strawberries
Toast
Orange wedges

Lunch

Gazpacho
Quick Tortilla Chips
Chili Salsa

Dinner

Salad
Spaghetti with **Spaghetti
Sauce#6**
Bread
Vegetable as desired

Dessert

Apple Bake

FRIDAY

Breakfast

Dorothy's Spanish Omelet
Toast
Orange slices

Lunch

**Mushroom Potato Garden
Gazpacho** (left over from
Thursday)

Dinner

Salad
Dressing: **Buttermilk Spring
Dressing**
Pizza
Mom's Spicy Eggplant

Dessert

Ice Cream Pie

TABLE 5.5. SAMPLE SHOPPING LIST

SPICES

1 jar	basil flakes
1 can	bay leaves
1 lg. can	cinnamon
1 can	oregano powder
1 can	oregano flakes
1 jar	rosemary
1 lg. jar	parsley flakes
1 can	black pepper
1 can	white pepper
1 can	nutmeg
1 jar	celery seed
1	garlic
1 jar	garlic flakes
1 jar	garlic powder
1 bottle	liquid garlic
1 jar	dill weed
1 jar	saffron
1 jar	pimento

CANNED GOODS

2 cans	evaporated skimmed milk
1 can	V-8 juice (unsalted if possible)
2 cans	tomato paste
6–8 cans	tomato sauce (large cans)
2 lg. cans	tomato puree
3 lg. cans	whole tomatoes
1 lg. can	tomato juice
1 can	canned California green chiles (chopped)
1 lg. can	green beans

TABLE 5.5 (continued)

MEAT, MILK, AND PRODUCE ITEMS
FOR SUNDAY–TUESDAY

Meat and Milk

6 lbs.	chicken backs and necks
¼ lb.	butter
¾ lb.	chicken breast
1 lb.	leanest ground beef
2 doz.	eggs
2 gal.	skim milk
1 qt.	buttermilk

Fruit

2 baskets	strawberries
4	grapefruit
4	oranges
1	watermelon
2 lbs.	bananas
2 lbs.	peaches
2	cantaloupe
2 lbs.	grapes

Vegetables

1 head	cabbage
3 lbs.	zucchini
1½ lbs.	bell peppers
5 lbs.	onions
1 head	celery
10 lbs.	potatoes
	salad makings
3	jalepeno chilies
3	yellow chilies
2	California green chilies
4	tomatillos
1 bunch	cilantro or coriander seeds

TABLE 5.5 (continued)

BAKING INGREDIENTS AND DRY BEANS

3 pk.	yeast
1 can	baking powder
1 box	baking soda
1 box	corn starch
½ cup	wild rice
1 lb.	lentils
2 lbs.	kidney or pinto beans
1 box	grapenuts
½ gal.	apple juice
1 can	frozen apple juice
2 lg. pk.	frozen blueberries
1 lg. pk.	frozen strawberries (unsweetened)
2 lbs.	frozen peas
1 bottle	lemon juice

MISCELLANEOUS ITEMS

1 pt.	wine vinegar
1 pt.	cider vinegar
1 pk.	raisins
1 pk.	Sap Sago or green cheese
3 pk.	corn tortillas
1 pk.	manicotti shells

MEAT, MILK, AND PRODUCE ITEMS
FOR WEDNESDAY–FRIDAY

Meat and Milk

4	chicken legs with thighs
½ gal.	milk

TABLE 5.5 (continued)

Fruit

4 lbs.	bananas
1 basket	strawberries
4	oranges
3	limes
1 lb.	apples
Some	other fruit in season

Vegetables

1½ lbs.	carrots
1 head	cabbage
1 head	celery
1 lb.	bell peppers
1	red onion
1	egg plant
Some	other vegetables in season
1 lb.	mushrooms
1 pk.	alfalfa sprouts
1 lb.	tomatoes
Some	salad makings

HEALTH FOOD STORE ITEMS

1 lb.	regular nonfat dry milk
5 lbs.	whole wheat flour
5 lbs.	brown rice
5 lbs.	7-grain cereal
2 lbs.	4-grain cereal
2 lbs.	rolled oats
1 lb.	bran flakes
2 pk.	Finn Crisps
2 pk.	Rice Cakes (unsalted)
2 pk.	puffed corn
1 lb.	whole wheat spaghetti
½ gal.	raw skimmed milk for buttermilk

Comprehensive meal planning also requires the preparation of some items a day beforehand. For this reason it is always good to make up a "calendar" of special events that lists those preparation jobs and when they are to be done. For our sample menus we have identified what these special jobs are, and when they need to be done. This calendar is shown in Table 5.6. Notice that even though the menus start on Sunday, as early as the preceding Friday morning you have to spend a minute starting a batch of "sour cream" (an excellent fat-free mock sour cream is on page 166). On Saturday, Sunday, Monday, and Wednesday, other tasks are called for.

TABLE 5.6. CALENDAR OF SPECIAL THINGS TO MAKE

FRIDAY
> Morning: Start **Sour Cream**[a] (or start it Thursday night, and check it a little earlier on Saturday).

SATURDAY
> Morning: Put on **Chicken Stock.**
> Make **Buttermilk.**[a]
> Afternoon or evening: Check **Sour Cream** and put through cheese cloth and into refrigerator; make **Chili Salsa.**

SUNDAY
> Morning: Check **Sour Cream** and put in containers for use.
> Remove fat and bones from **Chicken Stock** and store in 1-cup and 1-quart containers.

MONDAY
> Afternoon or evening: Cook **Chili Beans** (for enchiladas).

WEDNESDAY
> Early morning: Put on **Crock Pot Soup.**
> Afternoon or evening: Cook beans (any kind).

[a]These and other names in **boldface** are names of recipes in this book. They are not to be confused with commercial products of the same name. These recipes are fat-free. Commercial products are always high in fat.

CHAPTER 6

Your Weight-Loss Goal

How much weight should you lose? This important question depends on several factors and needs to be carefully considered. An incorrectly selected weight-loss goal can lead to disappointment and failure.

An unexpected discovery in recent years is that there are two kinds of obesity. What can be done to achieve weight loss depends on what kind of obesity* you have. The two kinds of obesity are characterized by the cells in the fat tissue.

Fat tissue is composed of billions of specialized fat cells. These fat cells have an important job to do. They convert sugar to fat, they store fat inside themselves, and they release fats for energy whenever required.

When your body needs to store away a great deal of excess fat, it has this choice: It can either store the fat in the existing fat cells, causing them to swell up and get larger; or it can create new fat cells, multiplying the cells in order to find space to store the excess fat. This is where the two kinds of obesity arise. People whose overweight is associated with enlarged fat cells form one type of obesity. People whose overweight is associated with the creation of brand new cells, resulting in a multiplication of the number of fat cells in the body, form the other type.

Cell multiplication occurs during the years before adulthood. When a person achieves adulthood, excess fat can be stored only in the existing cells. Weight gained as an adult causes existing fat cells to enlarge. No new cells are created.

---

*The word obesity is a technical term. It means excess body fat. It does not necessarily mean grossly overfat and it does not imply ugliness. Just as the person with 50 to 100 pounds of excess fat is termed obese, so is the person with only 5 to 10 pounds of excess fat.

During infancy, childhood, and adolescence, fat cells can increase wildly in number. A five- to ten-fold difference in the number of fat cells can occur from one person to another, and the factor that influences this number most is obesity. Thus, a person who was overweight in early life greatly increased the likelihood of increasing his number of fat cells.

Once created, excess fat cells are never lost. An overweight person with a greatly increased number of fat cells never loses any significant proportion of them. But he or she can shrink the existing cells.

The overweight person who is fat because of fat cell enlargement is in much the same boat. He or she can lose weight only if the fat cells are decreased in size. But this person's job may be easier. To reach normal weight, he or she need only reduce the size of the fat cells to normal size. The person with an increased number of fat cells can reach normal weight only by decreasing the size of the fat cells to a size *smaller* than normal. This is not an easy undertaking; in fact, people with increased numbers of fat cells have the most difficulty reducing.

"Adult onset" obesity is used to describe obesity that occurs after a person has achieved adulthood. "Adult onset" obesity is characterized by enlarged fat cells.

"Childhood onset" obesity is used to describe obesity that occurred before adulthood. It is characterized by an increased number of fat cells.

I believe that your weight-loss goal should be selected different if you have been overweight since childhood than if you became overweight only as an adult. Therefore, to set your goal, I want you, first, to decide which kind of overweight you have: adult onset or childhood onset. This may be obvious to some, and not obvious to others. You may need to look through photo albums or speak to relatives to determine the answer to this question.

Adult-Onset Obesity

If you have adult-onset obesity, you began gaining weight sometime after becoming an adult. This means that there was a period of time in your adult life when you were not overweight. It is this time period I want you to think about. Try to remember how much you weighed during that time.

Was there a body weight during that time at which you felt best? If you can recall a weight at which you felt best, let that weight be your *goal weight*.

If you cannot recall how you felt during those years, can you remember the least you weighed as an adult? If you can, let that be your goal weight.

If you can recall neither your minimum weight as an adult nor the weight at which you felt best, pick your goal weight using Table 6.1. This table shows suggested weight for a person of your body build and height. Use suggested weight plus 20 percent as your goal. If you are already not far from 20 percent overweight, set your goal weight at the suggested weight or at halfway between your present weight and the suggested weight.

Because suggested weights are based on averages of a lot of people, and are not generally accurate for individuals, the goal weight you get may not be completely suited to you, but it will be useful as a general guide.

Childhood-Onset Obesity

If obesity was a problem in your childhood, greater care must be exerted in selecting your goal weight. You will have to be careful not to pick a goal weight that is too tough to achieve.

It is likely that you have a lot more fat cells in your body than the average normal-weight person. As you lose weight, the size of these fat cells will lose weight too, by shrinking in size. But they won't shrink away to nothing. There are limits to how small fat cells can become. These limits, in turn, place limits on how much you can or should lose.

One way to determine how much you can lose is to examine your history of overweight as a child. What was the *lowest* percent overweight you were as a child? Were you ever only 30 percent overweight? 40 percent overweight? Your lowest percent overweight as a child can act as a guide now. If you could achieve that weight as a child, then perhaps you can achieve it now. Let your goal weight be

TABLE 6.1. Suggested Weights in Pounds,
by Height and Body Frame[a]

MEN   WOMEN

HEIGHT IN INCHES	SMALL FRAME	AVERAGE FRAME	LARGE FRAME	HEIGHT IN INCHES	SMALL FRAME	AVERAGE FRAME	LARGE FRAME
60	106	118	129	58	99	108	121
61	109	121	133	59	100	110	123
62	112	124	137	60	101	112	125
63	115	126	139	61	103	114	126
64	118	130	144	62	105	117	130
65	122	134	148	63	109	120	133
66	125	137	152	64	112	124	137
67	127	141	156	65	115	126	140
68	131	145	160	66	119	130	145
69	135	149	164	67	122	134	149
70	139	152	169	68	125	137	152
71	143	156	174	69	128	141	156
72	147	161	179	70	131	145	160
73	152	166	183	71	134	148	163
74	157	171	189	72	136	152	168
75	162	176	195	73	139	155	172
76	167	181	201	74	142	159	177
77	174	187	207	75	145	163	181

[a]Height and weight without shoes and other clothing. Adapted from Hathaway and Foard: *Heights and Weights of Adults in the United States*, Home Economics Research Report No. 10 (Washington, D.C.: U.S. Department of Agriculture, 1960), p. 51.

your ideal weight plus a percentage of this ideal weight equal to the lowest percentage of overweight that you were as a child. Here is an example:

Mary Carpenter has been overweight all her life. She now weighs 150 pounds, and because she is a small person, would have a suggested weight of only 100 pounds. Thus, she is 50 percent overweight. In checking her weight and height records with her childhood doctor, Mary found that at age 10 she weighed 100 pounds. She also found that her sister, Jane, at age 10 weighed 80 pounds and was the same height that Mary was at that age. Mary feels that she and her sister had about the same bone structure and that her sister's 80 pounds would have been a normal weight. Therefore, Mary figures that her 100 pounds at age 10 must have been about 20 pounds over normal. That's about 25 percent overweight. A goal weight for Mary today would therefore be her suggested weight (100 pounds) plus 25 percent. Thus, Mary's goal becomes 125 pounds.

Mary was lucky to have records to look up, and a good comparison in her sister, to determine a percentage of overweight that could be applied to find her goal weight. Perhaps you can figure out your goal weight by a similar procedure.

If you don't have access to this kind of information, there's another way to approach goal selection. Let your goal be the weight that is exactly halfway between your present weight and the suggested weight for you according to Table 6.1.

If neither of these procedures seems right *for you*, try one of the procedures indicated for the person who became obese as an adult.

Some Goal Hints

Goal weight will act as an objective against which you can measure your progress. It will also act as a reward for your patience and effort.

But goal weight can pose a danger, too. Failure to achieve it can be a disappointment that can wreck your weight-loss program. And the failure may not be your fault. It is possible that your weight-loss goal is unrealistically low *for you*, regardless of how it was chosen. Failure to achieve a too-low goal weight is only to be expected.

In the Live Longer Now program, the weight-loss goal you choose is only a means to help you. Since it is not possible to determine accurately a perfect weight for you, your goal can only be a direction in which to aim. The real measure of success in the Live Longer Now program is how closely you can adhere to longevity eating. Weight loss will take care of itself. The perfect weight loss for you might well be the weight loss the program actually produces in you as it acts over time.

CHAPTER 7

Two Weeks to Go:
Data Gathering and Practice

There are two weeks to go before you start the second phase of the program, your Weight-Losing phase. This chapter is about the first of those two weeks, and involves learning about yourself. The next chapter is about the second week and involves "adapting" to longevity eating.

In this first week of the program you will learn that managing things around you is more important in weight loss than managing yourself. You will select an ally who will help you in your weight-loss program. You will get a chance to keep a seven-day-journal of your food habits, which will provide you with a treasure-house of information about yourself. And you will do some "practice" eating of longevity foods to give you experience with your own longevity taste preferences.

Situational Management

Eating involves more than hunger. Eating is a behavior. It is a behavior done in response to cues around us. Things that cue eating, besides hunger, are things such as:

Time of Day:	"It's noon; time to eat lunch."
Mood:	"I'm depressed; think I'll have a peanut butter sandwich."
Activity:	"I always get the munchies while watching TV."
Food Cues:	"I wasn't really hungry until we walked past the ice cream shop."
Socializing:	"We always eat when we go out."

Cues like these, and many others, stimulate us to eat.

Seeing that our eating is to a great extent influenced by situational cues, we can, to a great extent, control eating by controlling the situational cues that lead to eating. Controlling situational cues is called *situational management.* Situational management to control eating and overweight is a complete reversal of the traditional means of weight control. Traditionally, weight control seeks to control you. Situational management, on the other hand, seeks to control your situation.

The two approaches are radically different. The traditional approach incorrectly sees overweight as something wrong with you that needs fixing. Situational management correctly sees overweight as something wrong with the situation around you that can be changed by corrective action.

Situational management is effective. It is probably the only effective weight-control technique among a dismal bunch. R. B. Stuart has shown that this technique is fully twice as effective in terms of the numbers of successful dieters as its nearest competitor. That is saying a lot.

But it is not saying enough. There are still a high proportion of failures even with this "most successful" of techniques. It is not hard to find the reason for these failures. Situational management by itself leaves unchanged the *kind* of food you eat. Thus, even when you are managing the situation around you perfectly, and eating cues are reduced or eliminated, you still must eat when hungry. And when you eat high palatation foods, your likelihood of overeating is great. No matter who you are. By the nature of the foods themselves. There is a built-in tendency to a certain amount of failure.

We will be using situational management in combination with longevity eating. This is a perfect combination. Situational management will help you stay within the world of longevity foods. Longevity foods will help you become slim. Situational management will be used during the next two weeks (the remainder of the start-up phase) as well as during the weight-losing phase.

In this first week, you will do three key things in situational management: (1) select an ally to help control your social situation; (2) gather key data by writing down what you see in your own eating situations; and (3) gain some experience in longevity eating situations by making and eating a few longevity dishes.

Selecting an Ally

The things that go on between you and the people around you make up your social situation. The important people in your social situation are the people you live with, the people you work with, and the people you socialize with.

Your social situation is full of food cues, things that influence how you eat. For instance, if your mate offers you a box of candy, several things may be happening:

1. Your mate may be saying: "This candy proves I love you and your eating it proves you love me." This is a strong cue to eat the candy.
2. Your mate may be saying: "You need a break, and eating this candy will be an enjoyable diversion from your everyday tasks." This is also a strong cue to eat.
3. Your mate may be saying: "If you don't join me in some candy, you are a party pooper." Another reason to eat.
4. The sight and smell of the candy itself provide still other strong eating cues.

Cues similar to the above may happen whenever neighbors, friends, family, or office co-workers involve you in food-related activities: going out for lunch, having birthday celebrations, going out on the town, coming over for dinner, and so on.

Because your social situation is a source of many food-related cues, it is important to gain control over it. You gain control by enlisting the aid of an *ally*.

An ally is someone close to you who is willing to help you in your weight-loss efforts by helping to build around you a social situation that will provide good eating cues rather than bad ones. A mate who is sympathetic to your weight-loss program could be an excellent ally. A friend or co-worker with whom you have daily contact, perhaps one also interested in losing weight, could be an ally. A parent, brother, sister, or other relative living with you could be an ally.

Here are some things your ally should be willing to do:

1. *Become familiar with longevity eating.* Reading this book or parts of it would be excellent.
2. *Encourage longevity eating.* For instance, by suggesting: "Let's eat at the Salad Bar where you can get an excellent longevity lunch." Or, "Wouldn't you like longevity lasagna for dinner tonight?"
3. *Offer plenty of support* for you when you show the correct eating behavior: "Congratulations on turning down the cake," or, "Hey, I see you took time to make yourself a longevity soup. Good for you."
4. *Respond neutrally when you goof up.* When you goof up, the ally's tendency is to criticize. But criticism of any kind is to be strictly avoided by the ally. The ally needs to remain neutral when you goof so that your attention will remain on your situation and not be diverted back to you, to your guilts and defenses.
5. *Help you set up your Action Plan.* In the next chapter we will talk about your Action Plan, a plan based on what you have learned about your eating situation from data you have gathered, and we will talk about the rewards you will earn as you meet the objectives in your Action Plan. Your ally will be helpful here.

Data Gathering

In this first week your aim is not to lose weight. That happens later and is described in Chapter 9. The object is not even to grow accustomed to longevity eating. That happens next week and is discussed in Chapter 8.

This first week is a time to gather data—to gather useful information. Therefore, you are asked during this week to eat exactly as you normally eat. Except for the experimentation with longevity food called for in certain paragraphs to follow, eat as you always do, so that baseline information can be gathered. Above all, DON'T DIET.

Two kinds of information on your eating situation are needed:

1. Information on those things in your situation associated with eating. You will need to keep an Eating Journal to record this information.
2. Information on those things in your situation not associated with eating, but things that you do a lot of. You will need to keep an Activities Journal to record this information.

Both journals are necessary to gather baseline data on your situation that will enable you to make your situation the best possible one for controlling eating cues and eating behavior.

Figures 7.1 and 7.2 are sample pages from Eating Journals, filled in for illustration for a man and for a woman. Each food you eat during the day, from the time you wake up in the morning until the time you fall asleep at night, should be recorded in your journal along with the things associated with eating: the time, the place, the company, and your feelings. These four things—time, place, company, and feelings—all can provide eating cues. Which provide eating cues for you, and how do they actually operate in your case? Your journal will reveal this to you.

Keep your Eating Journal current all day long. Write in the journal each time you eat, and make your entries under kind of food eaten and how much food you ate as accurate and specific as you can. If you ate ½ pint of ice cream at 2 p.m., enter exactly that information. Don't enter "dessert, medium amount, afternoon."

Figures 7.3 and 7.4 are sample pages from Activities Journals, also filled in for illustration for a man and for a woman. Complete your Activities Journal each night before retiring. Be as accurate and complete as you can. Try to account for every minute of the day.

By knowing about your activities, you will discover those "high probability" behaviors you exhibit every day that can act as substitutes for unwanted eating behavior. More about that in the next chapter.

Take a little time and care in setting up these journals. Use a

SUE'S EATING JOURNAL   DAY OF WEEK _Friday_

FOOD EATEN		THINGS ASSOCIATED WITH EATING			
Kind of Food	How Much I Ate	What Time? (Circle Time If Meal Was Involved)	Where Did I Eat? (Home, Work, Restaurant, Recreation, Etc.)	Who Was I With? Alone?	How Did I Feel? (Worried, Bored, Depressed, Tired, Mad, Etc.)
Omelet jelly Toast & butter	2 eggs, 1 oz. cheese 3 slices	8 a.m.	home	alone	rushed, anxious
milk	8 oz.				
Crackers Bologna Cheese diet cola	10 2 slices 2 slices 12 oz.	10:30 a.m.	work	alone	eating while on break
Vegetable soup Peanut butter & jelly sandwich cheese sandwich crackers diet cola	1 can 1 1 10 12 oz.	1 p.m.	home	with daughter	hurried, worried
fritos cheese cake iced tea	4 handfuls 3 inch wedge 8 oz.	2:30 p.m. 3:30 p.m. 3:30 p.m.	work work work	alone alone alone	guilty guilty
roast Potatoes Carrots onions coles law rolls w/ butter tea	8 oz. 2 cups 1½ cups 1½ cups 1 cup 3 8 oz.	7 p.m.	home	with husband and daughter	relaxed, lazy family atmosphere

Figure 7.1. Sample Page from Woman's Eating Journal.

SAM'S EATING JOURNAL   DAY OF WEEK *Friday*

FOOD EATEN		THINGS ASSOCIATED WITH EATING			
Kind of Food	How Much I Ate	What Time? (Circle Time If Meal Was Involved)	Where Did I Eat? (Home, Work, Restaurant, Recreation, Etc.)	Who Was I With? Alone?	How Did I Feel? (Worried, Bored, Depressed, Tired, Mad, Etc.)
Coffee	1 cup				
Bacon	2 strips				
Eggs	2, scrambled	7:30 a.m.	home	with daughter	anxious to get to work
Toast	2 slices				
Jelly, butter	2 tablespoons each				
Jelly Donut	1 large	10 a.m.	office	alone	anxious to get work done
cheeseburger	1/2 pound meat 2 oz. cheese	12 to 1	restaurant	with friends	talkative, happy
beer	2 12-ounce				
1 candy bar coffee	1 cup	2:30	office	alone	tired, depressed
Potato chips	10 chips	3:30	office	alone	tired
martini	1 1/2 oz. gin	5:30	home	alone	tired, concerned about work
Roast	1 pound				
Potatoes	3 cups				
Carrots	1/2 cup	7 p.m.	home	family	concerned about family
Onions	1/2 cup				
Coleslaw	2 cups				
Rolls - butter	3 rolls				
Beer	1 12-ounce				
beer	3 12-ounce				
bologna sandwich	2 (mayonnaise)	9 to 12	neighbor's house	friends	talkative, then tired
chips	30				

Figure 7.2. Sample Page from Man's Eating Journal.

SUE'S ACTIVITY JOURNAL   DAY OF WEEK *Friday*

TIME	DESCRIPTION OF ACTIVITY
6-6:30 a.m.	One-mile walk.
6:30-7:30	shower and dress; clean room; put away laundry.
7:30-8:30	Write letters, eat breakfast.
8:30-9	Drive to work.
9-10:30	work.
10:30-10:45	Read & eat on break.
10:45-12:30 p.m.	work.
1:00-1:30	Lunch.
1:30-3:30	work
3:30-3:45	Read and eat on break.
3:45-5	Work.
5-6	Grocery shop & drive home
6-7	Fix dinner with husband.
7-8	Eat and clean up kitchen with family.
8-10	chat with children, read.
10→on	Sleep.

Figure 7.3. Sample Page from Woman's Activity Journal.

SAM'S ACTIVITY JOURNAL   DAY OF WEEK _Friday_

TIME	DESCRIPTION OF ACTIVITY
6–6:30 a.m.	Read paper.
6:30 –7	Change plugs on wife's car.
7– 7:30	Shower and shave.
7:30–7:45	Eat breakfast with daughter.
7:45–8	Walk to work.
8–12	Dig through paperwork at office.
12–1 pm.	Lunch with fellows at office.
1–5	Finish paperwork.
5–5:30	Walk home; stop at hardware store on way.
5:30–6	Fix leak in basement.
6–7	Help with dinner.
7–8	Eat and help clean kitchen.
8–9	Read *Popular Mechanics*.
9–12	Play cards at neighbor's.

Figure 7.4. Sample Page from Man's Activity Journal.

looseleaf notebook, for instance, devoted entirely to the journals. Put seven sheets of paper in your notebook for your Eating Journal, one for each of the seven days you will keep your journal. Do the same for your Activities Journal. Rule off each sheet of paper in exactly the same way as shown in Figures 7.1 and 7.3.

Keeping these journals may seem troublesome, but don't give up. You only need to keep them for seven days, then you'll be done. And the information you gather will be well worth the effort. Most dieters who have kept a journal find it to be the most helpful and insightful part of their entire weight-loss program.

Some Practice Dishes

During the week that you keep your journals, experiment with a few longevity dishes. The only objective is to give your taste buds longevity experience before you begin full-time longevity eating.

Five practices are listed below. Do as many of them as you can. Do, at most, one practice per day. The dishes in these practices are very simple. The foods are simple, natural, low in fat, and high in complex carbohydrates and natural fiber. Pay close attention to the delicate flavors of these foods. Imagine to yourself the benefit your body is getting from them. Try to identify each taste, smell, and texture.

Practice 1

A Steamed Vegetable Plate. Choose an assortment of (3 or 4) vegetables you like. Suggestions: potatoes, broccoli, cauliflower, and onion. Use as much of them as you think you and whoever else will be eating with you will eat. Peel, wash, chop, and place into a steamer. Steam the vegetables until just tender. (Don't oversteam, they will get mushy and lose their flavor.) Sprinkle lightly with thyme and cumin. Serve and enjoy. A slice of sourdough bread and a glass of skim milk will go well with the vegetables and not detract from their flavor.

Practice 2

A Mixed-Bean Dish. Select an assortment of dried beans (about ½ cup each). Suggestions: Pinto beans, kidney beans, and garbanzo beans (chick-peas). Wash them and soak them overnight in 2 quarts of water. When ready to cook, add enough water to cover the beans well. Cook 15 minutes over medium heat. Add ½ cup each of chopped onion, chopped bell pepper, chopped celery, and sliced mushrooms. Season with oregano. Simmer 60 minutes or until each kind of bean is tender. Serve with a tossed salad and bread. Enjoy.

Practice 3

Broiled Fish Fillet. Select about a pound of fillets of any white-fleshed fish. Layer the fillets in a shallow pan and broil on one side until slightly brown on top. Turn fish over in the pan, sprinkle with about 1 teaspoon of paprika. Slice 2 medium onions thin and layer the slices over the fish. Pour ½ cup skim milk over the top of the fish. Return the fish to the broiler and broil until brown. Serve this delicious dish to 4 or more people. Accompany it with bread, skim milk, and a salad.

Practice 4

A Longevity Day. Below is an easy one-day menu you can make for yourself. Make and serve yourself each of these meals.

Breakfast
  Hot cereal: Stir a cup of rolled oats into a pan containing a cup of
    boiling water. Cook and stir a couple of minutes. Cover pan,
    remove it from the heat, and let sit 15 minutes.
  Banana: Slice ½ banana over the hot cereal.
  Flavoring: Top cereal with cinnamon and skim milk.
  Toast: Slice of toasted longevity bread (see page 212), or any
    acceptable commercial bread.
  Half grapefruit.

Lunch

Gazpacho soup: This delicious cold soup from Spain can be made up any time, refrigerated, and taken from the refrigerator ready to serve. Chop these vegetables finely: a green pepper, a zucchini, a stalk of celery, a garlic clove, an onion, and a couple of tomatoes. Place the vegetables in a bowl with 1 quart of tomato juice and the juice of 3 limes. Pepper to taste. Don't cook; chill and serve. You get 6 cups of soup, enough for several lunches.

Boiled corn on the cob: Place a couple of ears of frozen corn into a pot of boiling water. Boil until tender. Serve and eat plain; no spices required.

Salad: Make a tossed salad of lettuce, tomatoes, and as many chopped fresh vegetables as you have on hand. Make plenty; use the leftover for tonight's dinner.

Bread: Slice longevity bread or other acceptable bread.

Dinner

Spaghetti: Break up 1 pound of whole wheat spaghetti into a pot containing 2 quarts of boiling water. Cook rapidly until tender.

Spaghetti sauce: Finely chop 28 ounces of canned Italian plum tomatoes into a saucepan. Add a clove of garlic, finely minced, 1 teaspoon of oregano, and 1 teaspoon of garlic flakes. Cook rapidly and stir until thickened (about 15 minutes). Pour sauce over spaghetti and serve.

Bread: Serve plenty of longevity bread or other acceptable bread.

Tossed salad: Use the salad served at lunch.

Beverage: Serve iced linden tea.

Practice 5

Eating Out. Take yourself out to a restaurant and see how you fare ordering only longevity foods. Things to look for: broiled fish, broiled chicken, boiled lobster,* boiled clams, lettuce, baked potato, steamed corn on the cob, tomato and vegetable salad, sourdough

*Lobster is a shellfish. All shellfish were forbidden foods in *Live Longer Now,* due to cholesterol content. More recent data, however, has shown that the cholesterol content of some shellfish is sufficiently low as to make the food acceptable. Lobster is one of these acceptable shellfish. So are clams and scallops. Shrimp is out, however, and crab is marginal. See Table 5.3 on pages 71–76.

bread (made from white flour O.K. in a pinch), fresh fruit, tomato juice, steamed vegetables, steamed rice, and decaffeinated coffee.

Precautions: Remember to eat only a small portion of any meat, fish, or chicken dish, no matter how large a portion you are served. Check with the chef to be sure that no sauces are added to the fish, chicken, lobster, etc. Watch out for butter or sauces added in the kitchen to corn on the cob, baked potatoes, vegetables, rice, etc. It is sometimes difficult to convince the chef that you *really, really,* don't want any added sauces. (If your steamed vegetables come out soggy instead of crisp and tender, just remember the chef may never have cooked vegetables properly before in his life. His experience has probably been limited to cooking vegetables drowned in high palatation sauces. He's never had to worry about what the vegetables themselves taste like.)

CHAPTER 8

One Week to Go: Adaptation

Longevity eating is different. The difference between how you were eating before and how you will now begin eating separates the fat you of the past from the slim you of the future.

Because longevity eating is different from customary Western habits, it takes some getting used to. The second week of the start-up phase is an "adaptation period" designed to allow your body to get used to longevity eating. During the adaptation period you will concern yourself with sticking as close to pure longevity eating as you possibly can. How much you eat isn't important during adaptation; what is important is that you eat only longevity foods.

It has been our experience at the Institute of Health that adaptation takes about seven days. After seven days, longevity food will feel "right" to you and you will be able to enter the second, weight-losing, phase of the program.

You may begin to lose weight immediately, even during adaptation. Most people do. If this is the case, well and good. You are already losing weight and you haven't even started the second phase.

But, whether you lose or not, the adaptation period is vital. It is here that fundamental changes take place in your body.

Changes in Your Body

You will feel changes in your body during adaptation. You will feel the shift your body makes from a metabolism based on fat to a metabolism based on carbohydrates.

One important change is in the bacteria that live in your intestines. Your intestinal tract is richly populated with bacterial strains of many kinds. The same is true of the digestive tracts of all other humans and all species of animals on earth. These bacteria are important. They play a role in digestion. They flourish or decline depending on the food you eat. When you eat a high-fat diet, certain anaerobic bacteria flourish. When you change to a low-fat, high-complex-carbohydrate diet, these anaerobic bacteria die off (they are reduced 3000 percent in number) and other bacteria take their place.

Several investigators have shown that the anaerobic bacteria that develop and flourish in a high-fat diet produce cancer-causing chemicals. Vivienne Aries of St. Mary's Hospital in London showed that Englishmen, who have a high incidence of colon cancer, have 30 times as many of these bacteria as do Ugandans, whose incidence of colon cancer is practically nil.

Another important change is in the speed at which your digestive system works. On longevity food, your digestive system processes what you eat much faster than on regular Western food. Speed of processing is measured by what is known as "transit time." Transit time is the number of hours it takes from the time you eat your food until this food has been processed and is being eliminated from the body.

If you are an average American, you have a transit time somewhere between 50 and 75 hours. This means that the food you eat Monday at suppertime is still in your digestive tract all day Tuesday, all day Wednesday, and often all day Thursday.

Many investigators have found that the addition of unprocessed complex carbohydrate foods to the diet speeds up transit time. USDA researchers Kelsay, Behall, and Prather have shown that by merely substituting the whole citrus fruit in place of citrus juices, transit time in a group of subjects could be reduced from 52 hours to 38 hours.

Investigations of native population groups who eat longevity foods regularly demonstrate that transit time can be very short indeed. In his study of South African schoolchildren Walker showed that the transit time of these people averages only 9.5 hours.

Inferred from Walker's studies, and my own experiences at the Institute of Health, is that Americans who adopt longevity food habits will also have a short transit time, on the order of 9 to 12 hours. This means that food eaten at suppertime will be processed and ready for elimination by the following morning.

In addition to short transit time, longevity eating promotes larger, softer, and more frequent bowel movements. This is important. Anyone who has suffered from constipation knows how important. Not only constipation but the much more serious, and very common, disease called diverticulosis has been shown to be absent from populations that eat longevity foods.

In diverticulosis, the intestinal tract develops hernias (that is, unwanted pouches) along the intestinal wall. These hernias trap food being processed and encourage inflammatory damage to the intestines. Hernias are thought to be caused by the extra work the intestines have to do in order to digest Western foods. Western foods produce small, hard material for the intestines to process, and the intestines must work for long periods of time because of the long transit time associated with these foods. Under these conditions, the pressure in the intestines becomes elevated, and this elevated pressure causes hernias to develop. The large, soft digestive material associated with longevity foods leads to low pressure and does not produce the hernias of diverticulosis.

A further change you will experience has to do with your tolerance to fatty foods. When you don't eat fatty foods, your body makes an adjustment that makes fat less digestible. After this adjustment, you will probably find that a brief return to fatty foods does not agree with you. A binge on fatty foods at a fine restaurant might well leave you feeling nauseous and wishing you hadn't done it. You will then have developed an *intolerance* to fats. If you were to persist in eating fatty foods, this fat intolerance would leave you and you would be back where you started.

Finally, you will experience dramatic changes in your food tastes. During the first few days of adaptation you may notice most the *absences* that go with longevity foods. The absence of the taste-makers salt, sugar, and fat may give you a feeling of blandness or tastelessness. But as days pass you will begin to appreciate the *presence* of tastes that go with longevity foods. Your taste horizons will increase dramatically. You will replace the narrow but powerful taste experiences of salt, sugar, and fat with the broad but delicate taste experiences of natural foods. Interestingly, you may not recognize these changes for what they are. At the end of ten days many people at the Institute of Health have remarked: ''The dishes served during the last few days at the Institute are much better than those served the first few days." Actually, the tastiest meals are always served first. But they may not be recognized as such until taste adjustments have been made.

We all think that our taste preferences are best and that we couldn't possibly change them. Yet, an incredible variety of food is eaten by people around the world. Fish eggs in Russia, snails in France, fresh blood in Masailand, frozen blubber in Alaska, chocolate grasshoppers in Mexico, and filet mignon in the United States. All these things are delicacies to someone.

Tastes are learned. They are not inborn. New tastes can be learned, and old tastes can be unlearned. The adaptation period is a process of unlearning the old and learning the new.

The pleasure of eating is just as great with one set of tastes as another. You may as well adopt a set of tastes that will lead to a slimmer, more healthful you: longevity tastes. The payoff is well worth the effort.

How to Adapt to Longevity Eating

There are six parts to the adaptation process. They are as follows:

1. *Learning* more about the process that will be going on in adaptation.
2. *Planning* what you will eat and what you will do during adaptation.
3. *Drawing up* the paperwork needed to keep records on your successes during adaptation.
4. *Controlling* how food around you is handled.
5. *Eating* longevity foods according to your own plans. (This is the step that takes 7 days. The other steps are brief.)
6. *Celebrating* your success.

Ready? Then let's go through all six steps in sequence.

Learning to Adapt

There are three things to learn before starting the other parts of the adaptation process. These three things are: (1) the "K-cup" concept,

(2) the "caloric intensity of foods, and (3) the Baseline Food Plan used during adaptation and also later during the weight-losing program of phase 2. These three things are all related to controlling your food intake. The best way to start on them is to relate the following story about Mary Carpenter.

Mary Carpenter, who happens to be a vegetarian, is using Live Longer Now principles to lose weight. She has begun by setting up her daily diet this way:

- 3 cups of lowest-calorie foods like green beans at 30 calories per cup
- 3 cups of low-calorie foods like watermelon cubes at 50 calories per cup
- 3 cups of medium-calorie foods like peas and carrots at 80 calories per cup
- 3 cups of high-calorie foods like whole grain cereal at 150 calories per cup
- 3 cups of highest-calorie foods like pinto beans at 220 calories per cup

Thus, Mary is taking in about 2300 calories a day. But that's not important. In fact, Mary doesn't even know what her total calories are.

What is important is how Mary uses information on her food to control her weight loss. Mary finds out that on this diet she has not lost in a week's time. She weighs the same as before.

Mary makes a brilliant move. She decides that 3 cups of high-calorie grain foods is more than she needs. So she decides to cut out 2 cups of these foods in favor of adding 2 more cups of the lowest-calorie foods.

The volume of food she eats is the same, but she has obviously lost a lot of calories from her daily diet in this switch (240 calories to be exact).

In another week, although she has now lost ½ pound, she is still not satisfied. So she decides to cut down still further by cutting down on her pinto beans, from 3 cups to 1 cup, and substituting 2 cups of medium-calorie foods like peas and carrots. That's another substantial loss of calories from her daily diet (another 240 calories).

In the week after this change, Mary loses a pound. She is pleased and decides to make no more changes for the time being.

Notice what Mary did. Without really knowing her total caloric intake, and going only on her knowledge of which are the high-calorie foods, she adjusted her diet to one that was providing a substantial weight loss. And her quantity of food intake was unchanged.

Mary adjusted *cups of food* rather than calories.

You can do the same thing. And you don't need to be a vegetarian like Mary. But first you'll need to learn a new concept: the "K-cup" concept.

A K-cup of Coffee?

You may be surprised to see that the next few chapters are sprinkled with phrases like "a K-cup of cooked lentils" or "½ K-cup of milk." A K-cup is not the same as a cup, but it is very, very similar.

The K-cup concept is introduced to help you control food intake with an approach like Mary Carpenter's. The concept is introduced to allow for the fact that many foods don't have servings measured in terms of cups, but in other ways. For instance, fruit is measured by the piece, meat is measured by the ounce, and grapefruit is measured by the half.

But there is a great value in having a single measure that applies to all foods of interest to us. That single measure is the K-cup.

If the food is usually measured in cups, then a K-cup is a cup. If the food is measured in some other manner, then a K-cup would be considered a single-serving measure using this other manner of measure. Thus, for bread and most fruit, 1 K-cup = 1 piece. Because the Live Longer Now principles place certain restrictions on meats and fruit juice, we have: 1 K-cup = ¼ pound for meat, and 1 K-cup = 4 ounces for fruit beverages. For most other foods, 1 K-cup = 1 cup, sliced, diced, cooked or uncooked, according to custom.

Table 8.1 shows what constitutes a K-cup of food for many longevity foods. The table also shows the *caloric intensity* level of these foods, a useful concept to be described more fully later on.

Please notice that foods naturally group themselves at different levels of caloric intensity. We all know how this works because we are familiar with high-calorie foods versus low-calorie foods.

The K-cup concept is affected to a certain extent by caloric intensity. We have set a K-cup of plums at 2 plums rather than a single plum. Why? Because we would like a K-cup of one fruit to be about as many calories as a K-cup of any other fruit. Thus, 2 plums is a K-cup, but 1 medium apple is a K-cup. And a K-cup of either one of these fruits is about the same calorically: 60 calories.

TABLE 8.1. CALORIC-INTENSITY CHART*

This chart divides food into five levels according to the caloric intensity of the food. Foods in the lower levels have less calories, bite for bite, than foods in the higher levels. This chart also shows the household measure that corresponds to one "K-cup" of the food. A K-cup is usually 1 cup, but this is not always the case because some foods are not commonly measured in cups but are measured in other ways. Thus 1 K-cup grapefruit = ½ grapefruit, and 1 K-cup T-bone steak = 4 ounces. For foods (such as fruit juices) that are limited on this diet there is an advantage to defining 1 K-cup to be ½ cup or ⅔ cup of the food, as has been done below.

QUANTITIES SHOWN WITH EACH FOOD ARE THE HOUSEHOLD AMOUNTS EQUIVALENT TO 1 K-CUP OF THE FOOD. FOODS IN BOLD TYPE ARE FEATURED IN RECIPES BEGINNING ON PAGE 157

LEVEL 1. Lowest-calorie foods: 1 K-cup = 30 calories or less

VEGETABLES

For these vegetables 1 K-cup = 1 cup (sliced, chopped, or whatever is appropriate): asparagus, bean sprouts, beet greens, broccoli (raw), cabbage, cauliflower, celery, chard (Swiss), cress (Garden), cucumber, endive, green beans (including yellow or wax beans), lettuce, mustard greens, radishes, spinach (raw), summer squash (including zucchini, cocozelle, scalloped, and yellow crookneck or straightneck squash), turnip greens, watercress.

*Longevity eating requires knowledge of the composition of foods. The most comprehensive book in existence for this purpose is *Composition of Foods* by B. K. Watt and A. L. Merrill. This 190-page book is a must for every serious dieter. It may be obtained through the U.S. Department of Agriculture or by sending $6.00 to Composition of Foods, P.O. Box 17873, Tucson, Arizona 85731.

TABLE 8.1. (continued)

MISCELLANEOUS

Lemon	1 large
Mushrooms	½ cup, sliced
Popcorn	1 cup

LEVEL 2. Low-calorie foods: 1 K-cup = 40 to 75 calories

FRUIT BEVERAGES

Apple juice	½ cup	Orange juice	½ cup
Apricot nectar	½ cup	Peach nectar	½ cup
Blackberry juice	½ cup	Pear nectar	½ cup
Grapefruit juice	½ cup	Pineapple juice	½ cup
Grape juice	½ cup	Tangerine juice	½ cup

FRUIT

Apples	1 medium (¼ lb.)	Oranges		1 small (⅓ lb.)
Apricots	2 medium (2 oz. ea.)	Papayas		½ small (½ lb.)
Bananas	1 small (¼ lb.)	Peaches		1 small (⅓ lb.)
Blackberries	⅔ cup	Pears		1 small (¼ lb.)
Blueberries	⅔ cup	Pineapple		¼ medium
Cantaloupe	1 medium (1 lb.)			(medium = 2 lbs.)
Cherries	1 cup (15 cherries)		or	⅔ cup diced
Figs	2 large	Plums		2 medium
Grapefruit	½ medium (1½ lb.)			(1½ oz. ea.)
Grapes, green	1 cup	Raisins		2 tablespoons
Guavas	1 medium (¼ lb.)	Raspberries		¾ cup
Honeydew	½ medium (1½ lbs.)	Strawberries		1 cup
Mangos	1 large (⅓ lb.)	Tangerines		1 large (¼ lb.)
Nectarines	2 small (2 oz. ea.)	Watermelon		1 cup, cubes

VEGETABLES
(cooked, unless otherwise noted)

Artichokes	1 large (1 lb.)	Collard Greens	1 cup
Beets	1 cup, diced	Eggplant	1 cup, diced
Broccoli	1 cup, (½" pieces)	Kale	1 cup
Brussels sprouts	1 cup (7–8)	Okra	1 cup, crosscut
Carrots	1 cup, diced	Onions	1 cup, chopped
Carrots, raw	1 cup, grated	Onions, green, raw	1 cup, diced

TABLE 8.1. (continued)

Peppers, green	1 cup, chopped	Tomatoes, cooked	1 cup, packed
Pimiento, canned	1 cup	Tomato juice	1 cup
Rutabagas	1 cup, cubed	Turnips	1 cup, mashed
Spinach	1 cup, chopped	Vegetable juice	1 cup
Tomatoes, raw	1 cup, chopped		

SAUCES AND DRESSINGS

Garlic & Vinegar Dressing	1 cup	**Spaghetti Sauce #6**	1 cup
Perfection Salad Dressing	1 cup	**Spiced Vinegar Dressing**	1 cup
Spaghetti Sauce	1 cup	**Tangy Salad Dressing**	1 cup

LEVEL 3. Medium-calorie foods: 1 K-cup = 76 to 130 calories

DAIRY PRODUCTS

Buttermilk[a]	1 cup	Skim milk	1 cup
Cream Cheese	⅔ cup	**Sour Cream**	1 cup
Dry-curd cottage cheese	1 cup	**Yogurt**	1 cup
Egg White, hard cooked	1 cup, chopped		

BREAD

Lean Longevity Bread	1 slice
Pita Bread	½ pita
Water Bagels	1 bagel

VEGETABLES
(cooked)

Parsnips	1 cup, diced	Pumpkin	1 cup
Peas, fresh	1 cup	Pumpkin, boiled	1 cup, diced
Peas and carrots, frozen	1 cup	Squash, boiled	¾ cup, mashed
		Squash, winter	1 cup, mashed
Potatos, baked	1 (6 oz.)	Vegetables, mixed	1 cup, chopped

[a] Words in **bold face** are names of recipes in this book. They are not to be confused with commercial products by the same name, which are always high in fat. These recipes are fat-free.

TABLE 8.1. (continued)

FISH, CHICKEN, AND TURKEY
(Flesh only—no skin, organ, or fat. Weight is before cooking.)

Barracuda	¼ lb.	Oysters	¼ lb.
Bass	¼ lb.	Perch	¼ lb.
Buffalo fish	¼ lb.	Pike	¼ lb.
Butterfish (Gulf)	¼ lb.	Red Snapper	¼ lb.
Carp	¼ lb.	Rockfish	¼ lb.
Catfish	¼ lb.	Salmon (Atlantic)	¼ lb.
Chicken	¼ lb.	Seabass	¼ lb.
Clams	¼ lb.	Sturgeon	¼ lb.
Cod	¼ lb.	Swordfish	¼ lb.
Haddock	¼ lb.	Tautog (blackfish)	¼ lb.
Hake	¼ lb.	Trout (brook)	¼ lb.
Halibut (Calif.)	¼ lb.	Turkey	
Lobster (northern)	¼ lb.	(light meat)	¼ lb.
Octopus	¼ lb.	Turtle (green)	¼ lb.

SAUCES AND DRESSINGS

Buttermilk Spring Dressing	1 cup
Chili Salsa	1 cup
Versatility sauce	1 cup

LEVEL 4. High calorie foods: 1 K-cup = 130 to 200 calories

PASTA
(cooked)

Macaroni	1 cup
Noodles	1 cup
Spaghetti	1 cup

BREAKFAST CEREALS
(cooked unless otherwise stated)

Cream of Wheat	1 cup	Shredded Wheat, uncooked	2 biscuits
Grapenuts, uncooked with skim milk	1 cup	Wheat hearts	1 cup
Malto Meal	1 cup	Whole-grain cereal mixes	1 cup
Oats, rolled	1 cup		

TABLE 8.1. (continued)

VEGETABLES
(cooked)

Corn, kernels	1 cup	Succotash	1 cup
Limas, baby	1 cup	Sweet Potatoes	1 cup, sliced
Plantain, 1 foot	½ plantain	(or yams)	

FISH, FOWL, AND MEAT
(Flesh only—no skin, organ, or fat. Weight is before cooking.)

Beef, good grades only, not choice or prime	¼ lb.	Pheasant	¼ lb.
		Rabbit	¼ lb.
		Tuna	¼ lb.
Duck	¼ lb.	Veal, thin class, chuck only	¼ lb.
Goose	¼ lb.		
Halibut (Greenland)	¼ lb.	White fish	¼ lb.
Lamb, good grades only, not choice or prime	¼ lb.		

SAUCES AND DRESSINGS

Blue Cheese Dressing	1 cup	**Mushroom Sauce**	1 cup
Creamy Salad Dressing	1 cup	**Pimiento Dressing**	1 cup
Curried Pea Sauce	1 cup		

LEVEL 5. Highest calorie foods: 1 K-cup = more than 200 calories

LEGUMES
(cooked)

Beans[b]	1 cup	Lentils	1 cup
Blackeye peas (cow peas)	1 cup	Limas, mature	1 cup
Garbanzos (chick-peas)	1 cup	Peas, split or whole, dried	1 cup

GRAINS
(cooked)

Barley, pearl	1 cup	Rice, brown	1 cup
Kasha (buckwheat)	1 cup	Wild rice	1 cup
Millet	1 cup		

SAUCES AND DRESSINGS

Compromise White Sauce	1 cup	**Tuna Mushroom Sauce**	1 cup

[b]Includes red, Mexican red, pinto, black, brown, white (navy), kidney, calico, Bayo beans, and some other varieties.

In order to understand the K-cup concept and be able to use it easily, you must become familiar with the preceding table, Table 8.1. The table divides longevity foods into five levels according to how many calories are in a K-cup: from less than 30 calories per K-cup at the lowest level to foods of more than 200 calories per K-cup at the highest level.

With this table you can control your food intake by simple adjustments of how many K-cups of food you eat in each calorie level. Just as Mary Carpenter adjusted her food intake by manipulating cups of food. More about this later.

Caloric Intensity

Bite for bite, some foods have more calories than others. We say that the *caloric intensity* of these foods is greater.

Fats and oils are the most calorically intense foods. A cup of cooking oil contains nearly 1800 calories. Lettuce is perhaps the least calorically intense food, for a cup of shredded lettuce contains only about 20 calories.

The caloric intensity of longevity foods was shown in Table 8.1. This table divides longevity foods into five levels of caloric intensity as follows:

Level 1: caloric intensity = 30 or fewer calories per K-cup
Level 2: caloric intensity = 40–75 calories per K-cup
Level 3: caloric intensity = 76–130 calories per K-cup
Level 4: caloric intensity = 131–200 calories per K-cup
Level 5: caloric intensity = 201 or more calories per K-cup

Because the table contains only longevity foods, fats, sugars and other gremlin foods don't appear in it. Therefore, the highest caloric intensity reached is only about 250 calories per K-cup (split peas, for example).

The table lists individual longevity foods, but not longevity dishes. Thus, casseroles, stews, soups, desserts, and other dishes that are a *combination* of ingredients are not listed. But you will need to estimate their caloric intensity if you are to control your food intake. Table 8.2 gives rules for figuring the caloric intensity of foods not listed. For foods like lasagna, which don't lend themselves to cup measurement but are usually measured by the slice, you'll have to "guesstimate" how big a piece of the lasagna is equivalent to one cup. (For a lasagna 1 inch thick, a 3-inch x 4-inch slice is about the same as one cup.)

Table 8.3 summarizes the different levels of caloric intensity. Use it as a quick reminder of which foods have which level of caloric intensity, and what constitutes 1 K-cup for most foods.

The Baseline Food Plan

In the Live Longer Now Quick Weight-Loss program you have a Baseline Food Plan that is the same each day. This plan consists of the kinds and amounts of food that will give you the calories and nutrients you need every day in order to maintain your health.

Table 8.4 gives the Baseline Food Plan in detail. This plan has foods from all five levels of caloric intensity and includes cereals, grains, fruits, vegetables, bread, and dairy foods. It provides a total of about 1000 calories a day.

But there are foods above and beyond this baseline that you are allowed to eat at your own discretion. These are called *F*oods *L*eft *A*bove *B*aseline, or FLAB foods.

FLAB foods are the key to your weight-loss program. They are the foods you will adjust in order to achieve the right rate of weight loss. Adjusting FLAB foods to control weight loss is explained in detail in Chapter 9.

Your baseline food program stays the same. You don't adjust it. You do adjust your FLAB foods. You adjust them to suit your own taste and your own weight loss. Figure 8.1 illustrates this principle.

TABLE 8.2. FIGURING CALORIC INTENSITY LEVEL
FOR FOODS NOT LISTED

The Caloric Intensity Chart on pages 114–118 shows the caloric intensity of a host of individual foods. But the chart does not show caloric-intensity levels for composite dishes like casseroles, stews, soups, desserts, and many others made from several ingredients. Below are simple rules for deciding the caloric-intensity level of any composite dish, provided you know the ingredients.

RULE 1. FOR DISHES THAT CONTAIN NO GREMLINS, MEAT, FRUIT, OR FRUIT JUICE: If the highest-level ingredient[a] is also the main ingredient, set the level of the food at the level of the highest level ingredient. Otherwise, set it one level lower.

RULE 2. FOR DISHES THAT CONTAIN MEAT: Figure the level as in Rule 1 but figure 1 K-cup to be ⅔ cup of the food.

RULE 3. FOR DISHES THAT CONTAIN FRUIT OR FRUIT JUICE: Our only concern is heavily fruit-ladened dishes. Figure the level as in Rule 1 unless fruit or fruit juice is the main ingredient. In that case, set the dish at level 2 and figure 1 K-cup = ½ cup of the food.

RULE 4. FOR DISHES THAT CONTAIN GREMLINS: Figure the food at level 5. Figure 200 calories per K-cup. Thus, for example, one cup of ice cream at 400 calories is 2 K-cups of level 5 caloric intensity.

RULE 5. FOR SOUPS AND STEWS: Figure the level by using the rules above. If the soup is thick, use this level. If thin, reduce to one level lower.

[a]The "highest-level ingredient" means the ingredient that falls into the highest caloric-intensity level according to Table 8.1, the Caloric Intensity Chart.

TABLE 8.3. Caloric Intensity Summary

LEVEL 1. Lowest-calorie foods (30 or less calories per K-cup[b]) includes:

   1. Lowest-calorie vegetables like lettuce and zucchini
   2. Miscellaneous foods like popcorn and lemons

LEVEL 2. Low-calorie foods (40 to 75 calories per K-cup[b]) includes:

   1. Fruit and fruit beverages
   2. Low-calorie vegetables like broccoli, carrots, and tomatoes

LEVEL 3. Medium-calorie foods (76 to 130 calories per K-cup[b]) includes:

   1. Dairy products and bread
   2. Turkey, chicken, and most fish
   3. Medium-calorie vegetables like peas, potatoes, and squash

LEVEL 4. High-calorie foods (131 to 200 calories per K-cup[b]) includes:

   1. Pastas and breakfast cereals
   2. Beef, lamb, veal, and certain high-calorie fowl and fish
   3. High-calorie vegetables like baby limas and yams

LEVEL 5. Highest-calorie foods (Over 200 calories per K-cup[b]) includes:

   1. Legumes like beans and lentils
   2. Grains like barley and rice

[b]For all meats, 1 K-cup = ¼ lb.
For fruit beverages, 1 K-cup = ½ cup
For bread and fruit, 1 K-cup often = 1 piece
For most other foods, 1 K-cup = 1 cup, sliced, diced, cooked, or uncooked according to custom.

TABLE 8.4. Baseline Food Plan

These foods must be eaten every day. They are essential to provide necessary calories and nutrients. They do not change. The Baseline Food Plan provides only about 1000 calories. You are allowed food *above* this baseline plan. You control the *food left above baseline* in order to get optimal weight loss (see Chapter 9).

	Approx. Calories
1 K-cup cooked **GRAIN** foods (level 5): Brown rice, barley, millet, etc.	200
1 K-cup cooked **CEREAL** foods (level 4): Rolled oats, whole-grain cereals, etc.	150
2 K-cups **DAIRY** foods (level 3): Skim milk, skim cottage cheese, etc.	200
2 K-cups **FRUIT** foods (level 2): Fruit or fruit beverages	100
2 K-cups **BREAD** foods (level 3): Bread, rolls, pitas, etc.	150
4 K-cups **VEGETABLES** (2 K-cups level 1, 2 K-cups levels 2 or 3): Salad, beets, squash, etc.	150 to 250
TOTAL BASELINE CALORIES	About 1000

FLAB Foods: Foods Left Above Baseline. FLAB foods are under your daily control.

LEVEL 1 FOODS:	LEVEL 2 FOODS:	LEVEL 3 FOODS:	LEVEL 4 FOODS:	LEVEL 5 FOODS:
VEG	FRUIT	BREAD	CEREAL	GRAIN
VEG	FRUIT	BREAD	Baseline Foods: These foods are eaten every day to provide a base of nutrients and calories.	
		VEG	DAIRY	
		VEG	DAIRY	

Figure 8.1. FLAB Foods and Baseline Foods

FLAB foods can come from any level of caloric intensity. The choice is up to you. During your week of adaptation you will keep a close record of the FLAB foods you eat, but you will not try to control your weight. You are just gathering information that will help you during your weight-losing program later on.

The only restrictions on your FLAB foods are that they should include *no more than:*

    1 K-cup of meat (total of fish, fowl, or red meat)
    1 K-cup of fruit beverage *or* fruit (not both)
    1 K-cup of mushrooms
    1 K-cup of dairy foods

Other than these restrictions, FLAB foods may contain any amount of any longevity foods.

A Philosophical Summary

Keeping track of food in terms of K-cups has a distinct advantage for you. It is a visual process. You can usually tell how many K-cups of food you are about to eat with a measuring cup and a quick look. Calorie charts are not needed.

Your Baseline Food Plan gives you a simple foundation for good health. The food you add above and beyond that (your FLAB food) controls your weight. Your FLAB food will add appealing variety to your daily menu, but it won't add a large quantity of food. Most of your daily intake will come from Baseline foods. This makes keeping track of your weight program *much* easier, because you need only control K-cups of FLAB.

Controlling FLAB foods amounts to controlling the caloric-intensity levels from which you choose your FLAB foods each day. The Caloric Intensity Chart is easy to become familiar with. It replaces the concept of "food exchange," a concept used in other weight-loss books.

Food exchange lists are used to simplify calorie counting. And they *do* make calorie counting easier. But they are much more complex than our simple notion of K-cups of food of various levels of caloric intensity. They are more complex because they must include not only control of your calorie counting, but also control of the nutritional value of the food you take in. Because the Live Longer Now Quick Weight-Loss program is based solely on a broad variety of vegetable, grain, and other natural foods, and because the program incorporates a nutritionally adequate Baseline Food Plan, food exchange lists are unnecessary. You won't find any in this book.

Planning Your Program

Your goal during adaptation is to pass seven days eating only longevity food. To achieve that goal you need a plan. In fact, two plans: a Meal Plan and an Action Plan (a plan dealing with those inevitable moments of temptation when you are stricken with a compulsion to eat problem foods).

Your Meal Plan

Your Meal Plan begins with the Baseline Food Plan as a broad guide. It doesn't specify exactly what you should eat, just general requirements: 1 K-cup each of grains and cereals; 2 K-cups each of dairy, fruit, and breads; and 4 K-cups of vegetables in which 2 K-cups are Level 1 vegetables. What might such a meal plan look like for one day? An example baseline menu is shown in Figure 8.2. You're not required to follow this example, only the general guidelines of the Baseline Plan.

On top of your baseline foods, add FLAB foods according to your fancy. **Dorothy's Spanish Omelet** for breakfast, **Spinach Lasagna** for dinner, and vegetable and longevity cracker snacks at other times might be your fancy.

It doesn't matter how much FLAB food you place in your Meal Plan. It does matter that it is 100 percent longevity food and that you keep track of it in terms of K-cups consumed. (Page 129 tells you how to use a FLAB Control Card to keep track of FLAB foods very simply.)

Put your Meal Plan on paper. Write down on a sheet of paper what you will eat on Monday: breakfast, lunch, dinner, dessert, and snacks. Then, on a separate sheet of paper, do the same for Tuesday. Do the same for Wednesday, and so on for the whole seven-day

K-CUPS PROVIDED

Breakfast

Food	GRAINS	CEREAL	DAIRY	FRUIT	BREAD	VEGIES
1 cup cooked cereal		1				
1 small banana sliced over top				1		
1 slice bread, toasted					1	
1 cup skim milk			1			

Lunch

Food	GRAINS	CEREAL	DAIRY	FRUIT	BREAD	VEGIES
1 cup tossed salad (Level 1)						1
1 cup vegetable soup (Levels 2, 3)						1
1 cup skim milk			1			

Dinner

Food	GRAINS	CEREAL	DAIRY	FRUIT	BREAD	VEGIES
1 cup tossed salad (Level 1)						1
1 cup **Acapulco Brown Rice**	1					
1 cup broccoli (Level 2)						1
1 slice bread					1	

Dessert

Food	GRAINS	CEREAL	DAIRY	FRUIT	BREAD	VEGIES
1 apple, cut up				1		
TOTAL K-CUPS	1	1	2	2	2	4

FOOD TYPES: GRAINS, CEREAL, DAIRY, FRUIT, BREAD, VEGIES

Figure 8.2. Example of a Baseline Menu[a]

[a] You are allowed foods in *addition to* these baseline foods. Please see pages 124 and 137 for instructions.

adaptation period. When you are finished you will have seven sheets of paper and seven separate daily menus. Use the section in Chapter 5 entitled Meal Planning to help you if you need ideas. *The Live Longer Now Cookbook* may also be helpful. And don't be afraid of making a mistake and planning things you later decide you don't like or don't want to make. You can always change a Meal Plan. Also, be sure to plan plenty of snacks like vegetable sticks. These snacks can be carried with you wherever you go to be sure you are never too hungry—the last thing a dieter wants to have happen.

Your Action Plan

In the last chapter you learned to keep two seven-day journals: an Eating Journal and an Activities Journal. These journals contain records of how you ate and what you did over a seven-day period. Now is the time to put these journals to use.

There may well be times during the adaptation period when you are sorely tempted to eat problem foods. Under what circumstances will these temptations arise? Your Eating Journal will help you pinpoint likely temptation circumstances right now, in advance, before you even start the adaptation period.

Look through your journal for "hot spots." Hot spots are times of day (or special circumstances) when you are likely to overeat or eat problem foods. Many people find that a certain time of day is a habitual time for problem eating. It may be in the afternoon before the kids come home from school or late at night in bed that you have a hot spot.

A hot spot can also arise as a result of circumstances. For instance, you may find you always eat after or before a visit from certain individuals. Eating when driving, eating when in bed, and eating when lonely are common hot-spot circumstances.

Find your hot spots by inspecting your Eating Journal. Write them down on a piece of paper. Now you know your trouble spots in advance.

Hot spots can be controlled by doing other things that *you* enjoy doing at the times (or during the circumstances) when a hot spot usually arises. Your Activities Journal will help you here. Look through your Activities Journal and find those activities you do frequently. These frequent, or high-probability, activities are the best candidates to undertake for each hot spot. Write them down on a sheet of paper.

Your high-probability activities could be anything: telephoning friends, studying, walking, doing reports, or even watching television. Whatever your high-probability activities are, one or more of them will be suitable as a preplanned activity to undertake during your hot spots in place of eating.

Your Action Plan incorporates information about your hot spots and your high-probability activities into a single plan. Write your Action Plan on a single sheet of paper in exactly the format shown in Figure 8.3, Example of an Action Plan.

Be sure to place the sentence "I gain control of my eating when I do other things I enjoy instead" at the top of your Action Plan.

At the bottom of your Action Plan be sure to write the sentences "There is no penalty for failing. I will just reread my Action Plan and rewrite it if necessary."

Staple your lists of hot spots and high-probability activities to the back of your Action Plan and put it beside your bed.

MY ACTION PLAN

I gain control of my eating when I do other things I enjoy instead. Here is what I will do during my hot spots:

1. My Number 1 hot spot is: _____
    During this hot spot I plan to do this activity: _____

2. My Number 2 hot spot is: _____
    During this hot spot I plan to do this activity: _____

3. My Number 3 hot spot is: _____
    During this hot spot I plan to do this activity: _____

THERE IS NO PENALTY FOR FAILING. I will just reread this Action Plan and rewrite it if necessary.

Figure 8.3. Example of an Action Plan

Doing the Paperwork

One of the most important parts of this weight-loss program is keeping a record of your successes. To do this, you need to sit down and draw up the paperwork you will need for easy recordkeeping.

FLAB Control Cards

The FLAB Control Card is a seven-day record of your weight and the FLAB food you eat. During the seven-day adaptation period, you will enter information on your FLAB card every day. In the morning you will weigh yourself and enter your weight on the card. During the day you will enter the K-cups of FLAB food you eat on the card. Then in the evening you will calculate something new: your FLAB Index, to be entered on the card.

The FLAB Index is a way of letting you know how "hot" (in terms of calories) your FLAB foods were during the day. An index of 100 is pretty hot, and many dieters would gain a little if their index were 100 every day. An index of 50 is pretty chilly, and most dieters would lose if their index were always 50. Of course, you are not "most dieters." You are *you*. And you won't know what FLAB Index will cause weight loss or weight gain until you have kept track of it for a while. During adaptation, your interest in the FLAB Control Card is not in weight loss per se, but rather in data gathering. You want to gather data on how your body weight responds to FLAB foods over a seven-day period.

A sample FLAB Control Card is shown in Figure 8.4. In this example the dieter ate as few as 5 K-cups of FLAB food on Saturday and as many as 13 K-cups of FLAB food on Wednesday. The FLAB index ranged from a low of 52 on Saturday to a high of 104 on Tuesday. Body weight rose a little and fell a little, but over the week was unchanged. The average FLAB index for the whole week was 75.7.

A sample calculation for a FLAB Index is shown in Figure 8.5. On this particular Tuesday the FLAB index reads 93. How was this gotten? Simply by multiplying the number of K-cups eaten at each level by a multiplier, then adding the answers. The multiplier reflects the caloric intensity. The multiplier for Level 1 food is only 2, but it

FLAB CONTROL CARD

	FOODS LEFT ABOVE BASELINE (IN K-CUPS)					WEIGHT AND FLAB INDEX	
	Level 1 Foods	Level 2 Foods	Level 3 Foods	Level 4 Foods	Level 5 Foods	FLAB index (evening)	Weight (morning)
Mon	2	2	1	2	2	94	175
Tues	2	2	2	2	2	104	175¼
Wed	5	4	2	2	0	80	176
Thur	4	3	2	2	0	73	176
Fri	4	3	3	0	0	53	175¾
Sat	1	1	1	1	1	52	175¼
Sun	2	1	1	1	2	74	175
	x 2	x 5	x 10	x 15	x 20		

Weekly Total FLAB Index → Total: __530__
Average FLAB (total ÷ 7) → Average: __75.7__

Figure 8.4. A Sample FLAB Control Card

FLAB CONTROL CARD

	FOODS LEFT ABOVE BASELINE (IN K-CUPS)					WEIGHT AND FLAB INDEX	
	Level 1 Foods	Level 2 Foods	Level 3 Foods	Level 4 Foods	Level 5 Foods	FLAB index (evening)	Weight (morning)
Mon							
Tues	4	3	3	0	2	93	
Wed							
Thur							
Fri							
Sat							
Sun							
	4 x 2	3 x 5	3 x 10	0 x 15	2 x 20 =	93	

Weekly Total FLAB Index → Total: __93__
Average FLAB (total ÷ 7) → Average: _____

Figure 8.5. How to Calculate a FLAB Index

gets larger with each level. For Level 5 foods, the multiplier has grown to 20! A FLAB Index is easy to compute and gives you a nice measure of how calorically "hot" your food is each day. "Hot" foods put weight on; "cool" foods take it off.

Make your own FLAB Control Card exactly as shown in Figure 8.6. Use a 4 x 6 index card and rule it off as shown. The numbers at the bottom of each column are the numbers to multiply K-cups by to get your FLAB Index. (Figure 8.5 shows you how to compute a FLAB Index.) With practice, you should be able to do this in your head.

Weigh yourself at the same time each day, preferably in the morning before you have eaten anything or had any liquids (including water), and after you have been to the bathroom. Weigh nude or with the same clothes on each time you weigh. Be sure your scale is in good working order. (Check it against your doctor's scale or the scale at the YMCA.)

FLAB CONTROL CARD								
	FOODS LEFT ABOVE BASELINE (IN K-CUPS)						WEIGHT AND FLAB INDEX	
	Level 1 Foods	Level 2 Foods	Level 3 Foods	Level 4 Foods	Level 5 Foods		FLAB index (evening)	Weight (morning)
Mon								
Tues								
Wed								
Thur								
Fri								
Sat								
Sun								
	x 2	x 5	x 10	x 15	x 20			

Weekly Total FLAB Index → Total: _____
Average FLAB (total ÷ 7) → Average: _____

Figure 8.6. FLAB Control Card

Score Chart

Reward yourself with points for your achievements during adaptation. You may as well admit it: What you are doing during adaptation is heroic. And heroes and heroines deserve credit for what they do. You not only deserve credit for what you are accomplishing, you *need* this credit. You need it to give feedback and positive reinforcement to the new behaviors you and your body are developing about food. Therefore, I have provided you with a Score Chart (Figure 8.7) for you to record points you earn during adaptation. This chart gives you points each time you eat a "perfect" meal. (A perfect meal is one adhering 100 percent to longevity eating principles, as you understand them.) It also gives you points each time you defeat an urge to eat problem food. Record your points as soon as you earn them. Don't wait. You need credit right away.

Have you ever heard the phrase "Redeem your coupons for valuable prizes"? This is what I want you to do with the points you earn during adaptation.

Think of each point as a coupon. These are coupons you have earned. You can redeem them for valuable prizes. All you need is a catalogue of prizes and how many coupons or points are needed for each prize.

Have your ally help you make a redemption catalogue suitable to you and your way of life. An example might look like this:

COUPON REDEMPTION CATALOGUE

Coupons	Prize
5	20 minutes off to read.
25	Evening at theater.
50	New suit of clothes.
100	Weekend trip.

Your Score Chart will tell you how many coupons you have accumulated. You can redeem coupons as soon as you have enough for a prize or at any later time. Make a notation on your Score Chart whenever you use up points redeeming a prize.

SCORE CHART: Record all the points you earn during the week on this chart. Record them *as you earn them.* You score points for each perfect meal, perfect snacking, or perfect day you complete. "Perfect" means without problem foods. You also score points every time you defeat an urge to eat problem foods. Keep a tally at the bottom of this chart each time you defeat an urge. At the end of the day, this tally is your "urge score."

	1st Day	2nd Day	3rd Day	4th Day	5th Day	6th Day	7th Day	
URGE SCORE (Your Tally of Urge Defeats):								
PERFECT BREAKFAST? Score 2 points								
PERFECT LUNCH? Score 2 points								
PERFECT DINNER? Score 3 points								
PERFECT SNACKS through whole day? Score 1 point								
PERFECT DAY ALL DAY? Score 8 points								
TOTAL POINTS								
TALLY OF URGE DEFEATS								

Figure 8.7. A Score Chart

Controlling Food Cues

In Chapter 7 we talked about how things around you act as signals to eat. These signals, or cues, might be things people do, such as offering you food, or they might simply be the sights and smells of food.

An important step in successful adaptation is controlling these cues: getting rid of cues that stimulate you to eat problem foods and reinforcing cues that stimulate you to eat longevity foods. Your ally will help you by giving you positive verbal cues like "keep up the good work." And there are simple things you can do to improve other cues.

Make Eating a Pure Experience

Most people, and this probably includes you, combine eating with activities like watching television or reading. This creates a problem because these other activities become associated with food. They become food cues. If watching TV becomes a food cue, then every time you sit down to watch, you will get the urge to eat. You know what this is like if you have combined nibbling with TV watching.

You can handle a lot of eating cues all at once by making eating a pure experience. When you eat, eat. Do nothing else. Prepare yourself a place at the table, sit down, eat, and enjoy your food. Don't combine other activities with eating. Make this a firm resolution and stick with it. Having done this, you will have removed a host of problem-filled eating cues with one stroke.

Make Your Meals Attractive

Provide yourself positive food cues by making your meals as attractive as possible. Keep on hand at all times a plentiful supply of the freshest longevity foods. Serve longevity food in your nicest serving dishes, and make your place setting as pretty as possible. And even when storing longevity food in the refrigerator or on shelves, use nice-looking containers. The more pleasurable the eating setting, the stronger and more positive the eating cue.

Place Problem Foods Out of Sight

Sights and smells of food are food cues. It is best to rid your house and your environment of all problem foods and reminders of problem foods. Of course, if you are living with others, this may not be possible. But place problem foods out of sight: on the bottom shelf of the refrigerator, behind other things, and at the back of cupboards. Keep food in the kitchen rather than in other rooms of the house. If you have to prepare and handle problem foods for others, try to separate yourself emotionally from the food. If, as the cook, you *have* to taste problem foods, do as professional tasters do: taste and spit. Don't swallow. When cleaning plates, clean them directly into the garbage. Don't feel obliged to consume food the children didn't finish.

Problem foods enter your life outside the home too. Sometimes just driving by your favorite restaurant can be a strong food cue. So avoid that route if possible. If you work where a "lunch wagon" makes rounds during the day, be prepared. You might have a longevity snack while your co-workers indulge in problem food. Or you might shift to another work location when the lunch wagon comes around.

Only you know what your temptations are—and you are the best person to decide how to defuse these temptations.

Shop from a List

When you go grocery shopping, make a list in advance, and buy only the items on the list. This is especially important if you are shopping for others who are not eating longevity foods. This will tend to detach you from the food temptations you will encounter at the store, and keep your mind on the business at hand: successful adaptation. Another help is to shop right after eating, and never to shop when hungry.

Don't Let Yourself Go Hungry

Eat every meal every day. Keep longevity snacks such as vegetable sticks on hand for between-meal eating. You should not let yourself feel hungry or weak by skipping meals or by not having a snack between meals.

Eating Longevity Food

The biggest part of adaptation is to spend seven days eating and enjoying longevity food. You have a Meal Plan to go by and an Action Plan to take care of areas of temptation. These plans will be a great help to you, but they are not fixed in concrete. You can change them anytime you decide they are not working best for you.

And for goodness sake don't feel that you are a failure if you give in to an urge to eat a problem food occasionally. You won't get as many points on your Score Chart, but you're not a failure. You can gain those lost points back by *defeating* a subsequent urge. Maybe that same day!

If you do give in to an urge to eat nonlongevity food, look at it as an opportunity to learn something about yourself. Examine the situation that gave rise to the urge to eat. What were the factors in the situation that contributed to the eating response? Can you modify these factors so as to get rid of the cues that caused the eating response? Reread your Action Plan. Does your Action Plan help in this situation? Should your Action Plan be improved in some way?

The adaptation period is seven days long for a reason. It takes that long for your body and your taste buds to adjust to your new food program. Adjusting is not necessarily easy. For many people the hardest day, the low point, comes on the fourth day, and everything after that is easier. So if the going seems particularly tough on the fourth day, you are right on schedule. You have clear sailing ahead.

Celebrating Your Success

After seven days, you deserve a celebration. You have your own Coupon Redemption Catalogue (see page 132). At the end of the adaptation period, to celebrate your successes, cash in some or all of your coupons for your own personal celebration.

One word of caution: Don't let your celebration distract you from your goal of achieving a healthful weight loss. After adaptation, you will move directly into the weight-losing program, which is discussed in the next two chapters.

CHAPTER 9

Achieving Your Goal Weight

In previous chapters we talked about adaptation and other things having to do with the start-up phase of the Live Longer Now Quick Weight-Loss program. Now let's talk about phase 2, the weight-losing phase.

Your weight-losing program is a direct continuation of the seven-day adaptation program that you learned in the last chapter. The *only* difference is that now you will adjust your food intake so as to produce weight loss. This phase of your program will continue until your goal weight is achieved. The things that were important during adaptation are still important in your weight-losing program:

The Baseline Food Plan will provide you a foundation of nutritious food that will stay the same day in and day out. It will give you about 1000 calories per day: few enough to lose weight, yet enough to ensure minimal calories and nutrients for health.

FLAB foods, or "foods left above baseline," provide you with a variety over and above your baseline fare. FLAB foods hold the key to your weight loss. These are the foods you control. You control your FLAB foods by calculating your FLAB Index, a simple measure of how calorically "hot" your FLAB foods are. A FLAB Index of 100 is pretty hot, and if your FLAB foods came out with this high an index day after day, you'd probably gain weight. An index of 50 is pretty cold, and at this level day after day, you'd probably lose. FLAB foods are controlled by adjusting the FLAB Index to a level that is just right for you to lose weight consistently at a reasonable rate.

The concepts of K-cups and caloric intensity are vital in your weight-losing program. During adaptation, you learned how to measure your food intake in K-cups and you learned to measure its caloric value in terms of caloric intensity. These two concepts will now help you adjust and control the rate at which you lose weight.

Your Score Chart was kept to record your successes during adaptation. You also need it now to record your successes during weight loss. You score points for eating properly. These points serve as valuable feedback to you. They tell you that you are on the right track; and they are redeemable in valuable "prizes." You and your ally will continue the Coupon Redemption Catalogue. Each point you score on your Score Chart is considered a coupon, redeemable for prizes as a reward for your successes. Make a seven-day Score Chart right now as you start your weight-losing program; then a new one each week thereafter. Make improvements or changes in your Coupon Redemption Catalogue as often as you please.

The Action Plan you used during adaptation summarizes your strategy for handling food temptation areas or "hot spots." Continue to use it during the weight-losing process, making improvements in it whenever necessary.

Adjusting Your Rate of Weight Loss

How fast should you lose weight? As fast as possible, you might say. Right. And how fast might that be? How many pounds per week can you expect to lose?

The Correct Rate

Losing weight means losing body fat. But body fat is your stored fuel, and the only way it can be used up is to burn it up. For this, you have to eat less calories than your body actually needs. When you do that, to prevent you from dying from a lack of calories, your body merely draws from your stored pool of fat and burns fat for fuel in place of food. Over a period of time, you gradually use up your stored fat. You lose weight.

The thing to understand is that fat is a *very* efficient way to store energy. If you were to eat 500 calories less than your body needs to function, your body would use up only one-seventh of one pound of fat in making up for what you didn't eat. That's not much weight loss considering 500 calories may represent more than 25 percent of your entire daily food intake.

But it is enough weight loss. In a week you would lose one pound of pure fat. Melted, that would be enough to fill two cups with liquid fat. In a diesel engine that amount of fat could power a loaded semitrailer truck one mile down Arizona's Interstate 10. And in a year, that rate of weight loss amounts to over 50 pounds of pure dynamite fat.

Another way to look at it is that you didn't gain your excess weight in a day. Overeating by 500 calories one day, enough energy to drive a semitrailer truck, will only add one-seventh of one pound of fat to your body. That is truly an incredibly efficient way to store energy. It takes a long time to gain 50 pounds of excess weight. And it takes just as long to lose it.

If you lose more than a pound or two a week, you may be doing one or both of two things. You may be depriving your body of important nutrients and you may be losing water and lean body mass as well as fat. You don't need to lose lean body mass and you should not deprive your body of important nutrients.

Therefore, over the long haul, while your weight-loss program is in process, your rate of loss should be about one pound per week: an excellent and safe rate of weight loss.

Achieving the Correct Rate

Achieving the correct rate of weight loss is not difficult. You achieve weight loss by reducing FLAB foods, of which you have a daily knowledge. Your FLAB Control Cards, which you keep current on a daily basis, give you this knowledge. Figure 9.1 shows Mary Carpenter's FLAB Control Cards for the first four weeks of her weight-loss program, one card for each week.

Mary's FLAB Control Cards record both her weight and her FLAB Index. Her cards show that with a FLAB Index averaging between 66 and 76, she is achieving a weight loss of a pound a week by the end of the fourth week. Mary is right on schedule. She has successfully found a FLAB Index that is correct for her.

That will be your job now: to find the FLAB Index that will produce weight loss in you.

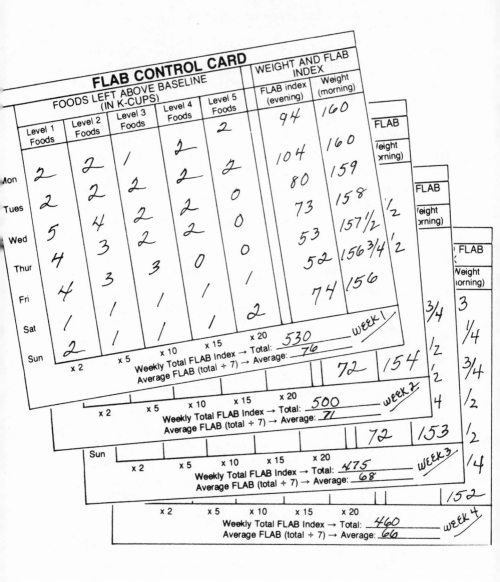

Figure 9.1. Mary Carpenter's FLAB Control Cards

As explained on page 112, the process of selecting foods with the right caloric intensity to cause weight loss is almost intuitive. Because you are weighing yourself every day, you will know whether you have lost weight in a week's time. If you have not lost, and if you have an idea of the caloric intensity of the food you have eaten over the week, you will know that you must reduce the most calorically intense foods in favor of less calorically intense ones. In no time, you will have yourself losing at the rate of a pound a week.

Getting Started

During adaptation you kept a single FLAB Control Card. This card will help you now. It will tell you whether you gained, lost, or stayed at the same weight during adaptation. It will also tell you your average FLAB Index over the week.

Did you fail to lose during adaptation? If so, take a look at your average FLAB Index. The way to begin losing is to reduce your FLAB Index. How is this done? Simply by eliminating some of the K-cups of food of higher caloric intensity in favor of K-cups of food of lower caloric intensity. This will automatically reduce your FLAB Index.

Your FLAB Index and your body weight, then, are the keys to your entire weight-losing program. As you watch your weight on a daily and a weekly basis you will see whether or not you are losing your pound a week. If not, you will simply reduce your FLAB Index.

Early Weight Loss

You may be pleasantly surprised to find that your weight loss in the first week of the weight-losing phase, or during adaptation, is substantial. It is common for a dieter to lose 3 or 4 pounds, and not uncommon to lose 7 pounds the first week.

You need to realize that this weight loss is not a loss of body fat. It is a loss of body water associated with stored carbohydrates. It is your body's natural response to eating less food. This high rate of loss won't last long. And it's not an important weight loss. It won't make you slimmer or prettier. It will just reduce the size of your liver and your extra cellular fluid volume a little.

Weight-loss programs that promise substantially more than a pound a week are trading on that first quick (and unimportant) weight loss. Losing body water and stored carbohydrates cannot long continue. And when the honeymoon is over, that "lost weight" will sneak its way back into your body, because your body needs most of that fluid and carbohydrate.

Reaching a Plateau

You may find that after weeks of successful weight loss you reach a point where weight loss tapers off. You are no longer losing weight. You have reached a plateau. What is happening?

For many dieters, there comes a time when the body begins to protect itself from further weight loss. It does this by increasing the efficiency of the utilization of food and by slowing down the body's Basal Metabolic Rate (BMR). The body may even go into a form of hibernation during sleep so as to conserve energy usage. The long and short of these protective maneuvers is that your weight loss stops.

If your weight-loss program reaches a plateau, don't worry. It's a natural phenomenon. Rather than reduce your FLAB foods still further, now is the time to increase your activity level. Reread the activity program in Chapters 3 and 4 and get outside for additional roving. Increased activity is a more direct attack on plateauing than decreased food intake and is your better bet.

If you plateau early in your weight-losing program, say in the first three weeks, you probably haven't found your right FLAB Index yet. In that case, go ahead and adjust your FLAB foods so as to further reduce your FLAB Index.

Your 18-Week Progress Card

It is vital to keep a record of your long-term weight loss in a form that clearly displays how you are doing. Your 18-Week Progress Card will do that. A partially filled-in example is shown in Figure 9.2.

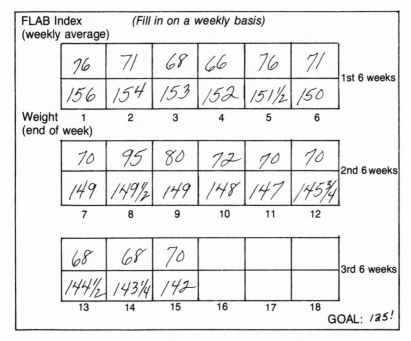

Figure 9.2. An 18-Week Progress Card

Fill in your progress card on a weekly basis from your FLAB
Control Cards. Keep it posted in a conspicuous place, perhaps on the
refrigerator door. The refrigerator is also a good place to post your
current FLAB Control Card. Whereas your FLAB Control Card will
fill up every 7 days, your Progress Card lasts 18 weeks before it needs
to be changed.

Weight Fluctuations

"Why is my weight going up and down?" On a daily basis, you
may find that your weight will occasionally rise a small amount. A
little up along with the down is all right. But on a week's basis, the
weight must go down if the FLAB Index is set correctly.

On a daily basis, there are things other than food that may cause a
weight gain. Your body has its own cycles of gaining, holding, then
releasing tissue fluid as you go about your daily life eating, drinking
fluids, and moving from an environment of one temperature and
humidity to another. The fluid that your body gains and loses has

weight. It may show up on the scales. But it is not fat. It is water. And it is lost as easily as it is gained.

Daily weight fluctuations will be minimized if you make sure to weigh yourself in the morning, either nude or with the same clothes on each day; and if you make sure to weigh before eating or taking fluid and after visiting the bathroom. Also, be certain that your scale is a good one, not subject to fluctuations of its own.

CHAPTER 10

Keeping It Off

It doesn't take any special commitment to read this book and become interested in the Live Longer Now Quick Weight-Loss program. But it does take a commitment on your part to achieve your weight-loss goal. And it will take a long-term commitment to maintain your goal weight over a period of years.

Long-term maintenance of your goal weight *is* your goal. Anything short of that is failure. Losing weight only to gain it again is both unhealthy and a waste of time.

Keeping your goal weight requires only one thing: sticking to longevity foods. The medium palatation level of longevity food assures you of a continuing mastery of your eating and your weight. And the high nutrient level of longevity foods, together with the protection from heart disease and other degenerative conditions that longevity foods have been designed for, assures you of extra years of zest and health.

The catch is that few people around you will be as committed to longevity eating as you are. In fact, most people won't even know what it is. Over the long haul this creates a problem. It places you in the position of having to maintain your commitment to longevity eating without the direct help of those around you.

Maintaining your commitment is vital. If it slips with the passage of time, so will your successful weight reduction.

To assure long-term commitment to longevity eating and guarantee that its importance doesn't fade with time, you will need some direct outside help. You're not alone. Everyone on the Live Longer Now Quick Weight-Loss program is in the same boat and has the same need.

To satisfy this need, I have established what I call the FLAB

Stoppers program: a little club you can join to give you continual contact with outside support for as many years as you need it. There aren't any meetings to go to. FLAB Stoppers is handled completely by mail by my staff at the Institute of Health. Members mail weekly data cards to FLAB Stoppers, and FLAB Stoppers mails back a personal progress profile along with other motivational data each month.

FLAB Stoppers computes the Master Points you earn while you are a member. Master Points are awarded as a direct measure of the work you do and the success you achieve during weight losing and subsequent weight maintenance. They are golden: hard to earn and invaluable to have.

You earn Master Points during weight losing at a fairly low rate (a few a month). You receive a bonus of 100 Master Points when you achieve your goal, and you earn them at a high rate (scores per month) for each month that you maintain your goal.

There is a superelite group of dieters: dieters who achieve 2000 Master Points. You cannot achieve 2000 Master Points without maintaining your goal for a long time: a minimum of 2½ years. Any member of FLAB Stoppers who achieves 2000 Master Points will be inducted as a Life Master in FLAB Stoppers.

There is nothing I want more than to have you become a Life Master in FLAB Stoppers. Believe me when I say that you can succeed only if you achieve your goal and stay there for an extended period of time. And the only way I will know whether you have succeeded is to have you join FLAB Stoppers so that I can get to know you and follow your progress.

I urge you to join. To find out how to join and what the costs are, send your name, address, and zip code to:

> FLAB Stoppers
> P.O. Box 2100
> Tucson, AZ 85702

CHAPTER 11

Easy Steps Anyone Can Take

I encourage you to adopt the Live Longer Now program in its entirety as it is explained in Chapter 2. But if you feel that this is too much for you, there is plenty you can do short of adopting the whole program. Any steps you take in the direction of the program are beneficial to both health and body weight.

In this chapter I enumerate eleven measures, any one of which you can adopt. Each measure is a major step into the program, yet each by itself is an easy step to take. I list the steps in order from easiest to hardest (as judged by most people). You can take them in any order, and you can take all or any part of them.

The more steps you take, the more of the Live Longer Now program you will have embraced. If you take all eleven steps you may be as much as 80 percent on the program. You would certainly find it straightforward at that time to tackle the program in its entirety. Thus, you can use these eleven steps as an introduction to the Live Longer Now program. After taking all the steps, turn to Chapter 2 and begin the program.

1. *Increase your intake of fresh whole fruits.* I am interested in increasing your fruit intake not because of the nutrient value of fruit or because fruit has any special value in weight-loss programs. My interest is to provide you with a food source that will tend to displace your eating of sweets to some degree. If not right away, then a little later. Because fruits themselves tend to be fattening, choose lower-calorie fruits like apples and oranges rather than very sweet fruits. Choose fresh whole fruits rather than canned, cooked, puréed, or juiced fruits.

2. *Eat more vegetables.* Eat more vegetables of all kinds: cooked

vegetables like broccoli, cauliflower, corn, peas, potatoes, zucchini, and beets, as well as raw vegetables like lettuce, tomatoes, carrots, celery, radishes, and cucumbers. Use spices to maximize delicious-ness. Avoid butter, oil, and other fatty sauces.

3. *Make your vegetables attractive.* When you serve vegetables at the table, serve them in your most attractive serving dishes. Arrange them in the serving dish as attractively and colorfully as possible. Use paprika, egg whites, or pimientos for extra color. Even when storing vegetables in the refrigerator, make them attractive. Keep them in attractive storage containers, and keep them fresh and appetizing. Buy them fresh frequently, and throw them out when they wilt, change color, get soggy, or in any way lose their attractiveness or zip.

4. *Decrease your contact with problem food.* Problem foods are the very high calorie foods so common in modern society: potato chips, cheeses, cookies, pies, cakes, fatty cold cuts, and so forth. By decreasing your contact with them around the house, you will de-crease your consumption of them. You can decrease your contact by placing them in the kitchen and out of sight. Don't keep foods in the living room, bedroom, or den. Keep them in the kitchen in cupboards or in the refrigerator. Keep them behind other foods, back in the far reaches where they aren't easily seen. Believe me, it's true; out of sight, out of mind. Out of mind means out of the stomach.

5. *Make eating a pure experience.* Frequently we eat while doing other things. This is a problem because we tend to associate eating with these other things. These other things become eating cues, and every time we do them, we have the urge to eat. When you eat, only eat. Don't combine eating with other activities like watching TV or reading. When you are ready to eat, first stop what you are doing. Then set yourself a place at the table, and eat your food there. Don't take leftovers to the TV or elsewhere to nibble. Either eat them at the table or put them away.

6. *Increase your awareness of fats in food.* You probably don't know how much fat you eat in a day. Few people do. But your intake of fat is nearly 50 percent of your daily calories. Fat is not only the fatty substance around your T-bone steak; it is also the oil in peanut butter, nuts, and olives. Butter, cooking oil, and mayonnaise are 100 percent fat, avocados are 80 percent fat, and whole milk is nearly 50 percent fat. Low-fat foods (under 10 percent) are vegetables, fruits,

grains, and nonfat dairy products. To increase your awareness of the fat in the foods you eat, read Chapter 5. Then, in the light of what you have learned from Chapter 5, try to determine which foods in your diet are especially high in fat and which are especially low.

7. *Eat more nonfat dairy products.* As a first step in the reduction of your fat intake, rather than cut something out of your diet, do the opposite: step-up your intake of nonfat dairy products. This includes nonfat milk, nonfat yogurt, and nonfat cottage cheeses (dry-curd cottage cheese or hoop cheese). Next, cut down whole milk and regular yogurt. Low-fat milk, low-fat yogurt, and low-fat cottage cheeses are O.K. as a compromise at first. But because low-fat dairy products are still relatively high in fat, the transition must ultimately be to nonfat products.

8. *Decrease your usage of added fat and salt.* Fats and salts are added to foods in the kitchen and at the table. You can cut down on these added problem foods easily. It is usually unnecessary to cook foods in oil or fat. For instance, vegetables sautéed in butter give you a dish that can best be described as butter with vegetable flavoring. Vegetables can be sautéed in water over a high flame and the result is deliciously cooked vegetables, not butter. Butter and oils are added at the table on bread, over vegetables, in salads, and so on. These additions are not necessary to bring out the flavor of the food. In fact they usually hide flavor behind the additives' own strong odors and tastes. Simply stop adding them, or at least reduce their quantity. Adding salt at the cookpot and at the table also can be reduced. Food value is not enhanced by salt. In fact, salt is harmful to your body. You will miss salt at first. You will not be accustomed to the presence of subtle tastes in unsalted foods. But you will quickly become used to real flavors and then won't miss the saltiness to which you are now habituated.

9. *Increase grains and cereals.* Eat more whole-grain foods: whole-grain bread, whole-grain spaghetti, and whole-grain noodles. Eat more brown rice, barley, and millet. Eat whole-grain cereals for breakfast with sliced banana, skim milk, and cinnamon as topping. You may need to find these foods in your local health food store. They are becoming increasingly available, however, in super-markets. Eat these foods without added salt, fats, oils, or sweeteners of any kind. These grain and cereal foods provide you with an

abundant supply of calories, natural fiber, slowly absorbed complex carbohydrates, and vitamins and minerals. They are low in fat but have plenty of protein and complex carbohydrate.

10. *Cut down on cheeses, nuts, and fatty meats.* With added cereals, fruits, and vegetables in your diet, you will find no difficulty in reducing your intake of the especially fatty foods: cheeses, nuts, and fatty meats. Fatty meats include cold cuts, sausage, bacon, and hotdogs. Fatty meats also include choice and prime cuts of beef and lamb, and fatty hamburger. But good gradè beef or lamb, and the leanest hamburger, present less of a problem. All cheeses are high in fat: 60–80 percent. And all nuts except chestnuts are high in fat: 70 percent or so.

11. *Decrease sweets.* Because you have access to fruit, cutting down on sweets will be less of a problem. Remember, sweets include not only candy, cake, pies, and other desserts made from sugar, but also honey, syrup, molasses, and all foods made from or with these ingredients. In cutting down on sweets it is helpful to keep them out of the house or at least out of sight as much as possible. It is also helpful to eat plenty of the less calorically intense foods, particularly grain foods, to provide a source of ''safe'' carbohydrates to replace those ''unsafe'' carbohydrates you are cutting out by reducing sweets.

The eleven steps are all excellent halfway measures to adopt. Pick and choose among them. Take those steps that seem easiest for you, and add others later. Perhaps you will soon be a long way along the road to longevity eating.

Below is a summary of the above eleven steps, for easy reference.

Summary of Eleven Easy Steps You Can Take

1. Increase your intake of fresh whole fruits.
2. Eat more vegetables.
3. Make your vegetables attractive.
4. Decrease your contact with problem foods.
5. Make eating a pure experience.
6. Increase your awareness of fats in food.

7. Eat more nonfat dairy products.
8. Decrease your usage of added fat and salt.
9. Increase grains and cereals.
10. Cut down on fatty meats, cheeses, and nuts.
11. Decrease sweets.

What to Do Away from Home

At a Restaurant

Here are some hints for when you are eating out:
Select a fish entrée and have it broiled without sauce. Use lemon juice in place of sauce. Don't feel obligated to eat the whole serving. Leave as much as you can on your plate. You're not wasting money, you are saving health.

Double up on lettuce, tomatoes, and baked potatoes. Take them all without dressing, but ask for lemon for the lettuce and tomatoes, and skim milk to moisturize the baked potatoes. Use pepper or other spices to top off the potato and salad.

Favor skim milk or tomato juice as your beverage in place of more fattening or stimulating beverages. Choose sourdough bread when it's available, and for goodness sake eat it plain, without butter, so you can enjoy the old-fashioned frontier flavor that sourdough possesses.

Choose fresh whole fruit for dessert.

At Work

Figure on packing a lunch to take to work with you. Eating your lunch day in and day out at a restaurant will not be satisfactory. No matter how hard it is to "brown bag it" on your job, give it a try. Very rare is the job that is totally incompatible with the brown bag. Even airline pilots on the Live Longer Now program have successfully switched to packing their own food to bring with them to work. This is quite a feat since an airplane pilot may have to be confined to an aircraft or airport for as long as 24 or 48 hours at a stretch.

Anything you can have for dinner can be packed as a lunch. If you have access to a microwave oven in your lunch area, you can simply fill up plastic containers with last night's leftovers right out of the refrigerator. Heat them in the microwave and you have a hot meal with very little effort. If you don't have a microwave, do any desired heating before you leave for work and keep the food hot until lunch in thermos bottles.*

Soup, stew, lasagna, spaghetti, or vegetable dishes make excellent hot dishes for lunch. Add bread slices, tossed salad in a plastic container, and fruit for dessert, and you have a meal that will be delicious and satisfying. And it will be just as easy to prepare and eat as the standard lunch of sandwiches. The only difference is that you will need to take your containers home with you to be washed and reused. This is a small inconvenience for such an excellent meal.

People ask me what kind of longevity sandwiches can be prepared. Since a sandwich is any food that strikes your fancy, stuck between two pieces of bread, you can make any kind of sandwich you want, so long as the food you stick between the slices of bread is longevity food.

Unfortunately the sandwich foods with which you are familiar are almost always problem foods: cheeses, cold cuts, mayonnaise spreads, butter, bacon, peanut butter, jelly, etc. And a lettuce, tomato, and onion sandwich might not seem like a real sandwich to you.

You may ask if there is some way to make a sandwich that tastes like one of our old favorites, like a tuna salad sandwich for example, but is free of problem foods. The answer is no, not to my knowledge. There is no way that longevity foods can be made to give you the same tastes and effects that problem foods do. Only problem foods can do that.

I have learned over the years that the secret to longevity eating is to allow yourself to develop new tastes so that longevity foods are what you prefer rather than to search for ways to make longevity foods conform to your old tastes. With a few exceptions, it is impossible to

*I should point out that longevity dishes differ from dishes containing problem foods that need to be served hot. Many problem foods are palatable only when served hot because their high grease content makes them impossible to choke down unless the grease is hot and liquid. Low-fat longevity dishes can usually be enjoyed cold as well as hot. Thus the need to heat leftovers is not nearly so critical on the Live Longer Now program.

create longevity foods that look, smell, and taste like the problem foods that are so familiar to us.

Dinner at a Friend's House

What do you do when you are invited to dinner at a friend's house? Be totally open and frank about your new eating program. Tell your friend that you are on a special program and that you are committed firmly to sticking to it. While you cannot expect your friends to prepare Live Longer Now meals for you, you can expect them to understand your right to eat in the manner you know is best for you. Most people are anxious to be helpful and will try to accommodate your needs in some small way.

You can expect, however, that most attempts to accommodate your needs will fall short. You can expect to hear things like: "Why you can eat *this* cake. I made it with honey instead of sugar and I used only margarine, not butter, so it is cholesterol free." Of course this well-meaning effort is still totally off target because honey is as much a problem as sugar, and margarine is 100% fat, just like butter.

It is very likely that the only way you will be able to stay on the Live Longer Now diet when you eat at a friend's is to pass up some of what is served. To be able to do this, your convictions must be firm. It will help if you let your friend know in advance that you may need to pass up some of the offerings, and it will certainly help if you assure your friend that your friendship needn't suffer because you will be eating differently. You and your friend may both decide on something other than a dinner to accomplish the socialization desired.

APPENDIX 1

Composition of Foods

If this book has a central theme, it is that knowledge of what food is composed of and the application of this knowledge to how you eat is the key to success in losing weight. In addition to what you have learned about the composition of foods from this book, you will need to know about other common foods and what they are made of in terms of fat, protein, carbohydrate, and other nutrients.

Without question, the most authoritative and comprehensive book on what foods are made of is *Composition of Foods*, put out by the U.S. Department of Agriculture, and authored by B. K. Watt and A. L. Merrill. This classic gives the vitamin, mineral, fat, carbohydrate, protein, and cholesterol content of literally thousands of common foods. Everyone interested in weight control or health should get a copy of this book. It is easy to use, it is informative, and it is fun to browse through. (See footnote on page 114 for information on ordering.)

APPENDIX 2

Roving and Food

As we have said elsewhere in this book, weight loss is controlled not only by how much you eat, but also by how much you exercise. When you eat, you add calories to your body's stores. When you exercise, you use up calories. If you use up more calories than you store, then in time you will lose weight.

Exercise acts in the opposite direction. It burns up the energy your food consumption banks. Thus, food eaten can be counteracted by the exercise you do.

This is a truly fascinating proposition for most overweight people. It implies that food indulgence can be atoned for by direct means: exercise. It implies that if I eat too much lasagna, I can escape the consequences of this indulgence by extra activity.

And this is true. For every quantity of any food you eat, there is an equivalent quantity of some exercise that will counteract the fat-producing effect of the food.

The food we eat in the Live Longer Now program is measured in K-cups of food. And the exercise we take is roving, in the form of walking, jogging, or running. Table A.1 shows the roving equivalent of different quantities of food. It shows you exactly how much exercise will counteract a given quantity of food.

For instance, the table shows that a little under ½ hour (28 minutes) of walking at 4 miles per hour (a very brisk walk) is worth a K-cup of the most calorically intense food in longevity eating, Level 5 food. And a little over ½ hour of running (34 minutes) would use up 2 K-cups of Level 5 food.

The table is interesting and informative, but it is not intended to imply that every K-cup of food you eat has to be counteracted by some amount of roving. Not only would this be unnecessary, it would be impossible. There would be no energy left for ordinary metabolism.

The table has its value because it shows you that the exercise you take directly affects the fat your body stores. Thus, slowing down the storing of fat can be done in either of two ways: eating less K-cups of food or taking more roving exercise. If you want to know how much exercise you would need to get the same effect as reducing your food intake by 1 K-cup at a certain level, Table A.1 will tell you.

TABLE A.1. ROVING EQUIVALENT OF 1 K-CUP OF FOOD

	Approximate Food Energy	Roving		
		Walking (4 miles/hour)	Jogging (6 miles/hour)	Running (8 miles/hour)
	CALORIES	MINUTES		
Level 1 (1 K-cup): Lowest-calorie vegetables like lettuce and zucchini	20	3	2	1
Level 2 (1 K-cup): Fruit and fruit beverages. Low-calorie vegetables like broccoli, carrots, and tomatoes	60	8	6	5
Level 3 (1 K-cup): Nonfat dairy products. Bread. Turkey, chicken, most fish. Medium-calorie vegetables like peas, potatoes, and squash	100	12	10	8
Level 4 (1 K-cup): Pastas and breakfast cereals. Beef, lamb, veal, and higher-calorie fowl and fish. High-calorie vegetables like baby limas and yams	175	22	18	13
Level 5 (1 K-cup): Legumes like beans and lentils. Grains like barley and rice	220	28	22	17

APPENDIX 3

Weight-Losing Recipes

These recipes have been selected for their value in weight loss. Some of them are from the *Live Longer Now Cookbook* (some have been changed slightly) and some are new recipes developed at the Institute of Health since publication of the cookbook. All are delicious and worth trying. (For comprehensive instructions on longevity cooking, including hundreds of additional recipes and helpful hints, the *Live Longer Now Cookbook* is a must.)

Throughout this book, whenever a reference is made by name to one of these recipes, the reference is in **boldface** type. A title index is included at the back of the book so that you will be able to locate any recipe quickly.

Three staple cheeses are used frequently in these recipes: dry-curd cottage cheese, St. Otto's brand cheese, and Sap Sago cheese. Dry-curd cottage cheese is the common name used for any cottage cheese made from 100 percent skim milk. (Safeway markets throughout the United States carry it.) It is sometimes pressed loosely into blocks and sold under the name "hoop cheese." St. Otto's cheese is a low-fat (less than 15 percent total calories from fat) sliceable cheese. Any comparable cheese may be used. But be wary. Cheeses advertised as part-skim-milk cheeses are usually over 50 percent fat. Sap Sago cheese is a 100 percent skim-milk cheese that is hard and can be grated into a Parmesan-like powder. It is green in color and is sold in small cone-shaped bricks about the size of a salt shaker. Use it, grated, as a flavoring for soups, casseroles, and sauces.

I use the convention throughout these recipes that pepper means black pepper, and that the ingredients in parentheses are optional ingredients.

For your convenience, I have indicated the caloric-intensity level of each recipe. See page 119 for a complete explanation of this very important concept.

BREAKFAST ITEMS

DOROTHY'S SPANISH OMELETTE
Level 3
(1 K-cup = 1 cup)

½ cup chopped green pepper
¼ cup chopped onion
1 tablespoon garlic juice
1 canned California green
  chili, chopped
½ small tomato, squeezed of
  juice and chopped

2 teaspoons chopped
  pimiento
6 egg whites
Pinch of saffron
½ cup grated St. Otto's cheese
(Chili Salsa)

In skillet, sauté green pepper and onion in garlic juice and 2 table-spoons water. Add chopped chili, tomato, and pimiento, and boil off remaining liquid. Combine egg whites and saffron and beat to soft peaks. Fold cheese into egg whites, followed by the contents of the skillet. Return to skillet and fry until eggs are set, turning to avoid scorching. Pour off any water rendered during cooking. Serve topped with chili salsa if desired. Serves 4.

BREAKFAST BAGELS
Level 3
(1 K-cup = ½ bagel)

Use those bagels in the freezer for a quick, popular breakfast.

6 **Water Bagels**
½ pound St. Otto's cheese
2 medium-to-large tomatoes
1 medium sweet red onion, sliced

Split each bagel into 2 circular half-bagels. Lay bagel halves, cut face up, on broiler pan. Slice cheese thinly, and cover each bagel with cheese slices. Slice each tomato into 6 slices. Lay one tomato slice and one onion slice on each bagel. Broil until cheese melts. Serves 6.

TOASTED WHEAT BERRY CEREAL
Level 4
(1 K-cup = 1 cup)

1 cup wheat berries (whole   2 cups water
  dried wheat kernels)   Skim milk

Toast wheat berries in Teflon skillet over moderate-to-high heat until berries spin, pop, and begin to brown. Combine with water in saucepan, cover, and simmer 45 minutes. Serve with skim milk. Serves 4.

STEEL-CUT OATMEAL
Level 4
(1 K-cup = 1 cup)

Oatmeal can be prepared in a variety of ways, and they're all good. This recipe uses long, slow cooking and steel-cut oats (each individual oat cut into about 3 pieces by blade-fitted steel rollers) to get a delightful creamy-style oatmeal.

⅔ cup steel-cut oats   Freshly ground nutmeg
 2 cups boiling water   Skim milk
Cinnamon

Add oats to boiling water, cover, and simmer 40 minutes over very low heat. Top with cinnamon and nutmeg. Serve with skim milk. Serves 4.

YOGURT CREPES
Level 3
(1 K-cup = 2 crepes)

3 egg whites   ¾ cup skim milk
½ cup **Yogurt**   ¾ cup flour

Beat egg whites and yogurt until foamy. Beat in milk, then flour.
Spoon onto hot Teflon griddle, spreading out into thin pancakes.
Turn as soon as spatula will slide under pancake without sticking.
Makes 16 crepes.

VELVETY PANCAKES
Level 3
(1 K-cup = 2 pancakes)

1 teaspoon baking powder   2 egg whites
1 cup whole wheat flour   1½ cups evaporated skim milk

Combine baking powder and flour. Beat egg whites to soft peaks,
then add milk and beat again. Combine wet and dry mixtures and stir
lightly. Teflon-fry pancakes on both sides. Top with a fruit sauce.
Makes 12 to 14 pancakes.

APPETIZERS

GARDEN BASKET
Level 1
(1 K-cup = 1 cup)

Served without a dip, this appetizer is light as Spring and deliciously attractive. Make a spray arrangement of long carrot and celery sticks (leaves remaining on some of the celery sticks) in an attractive napkin-lined bread basket. Place radish rosettes over the carrots and celery to give the impression of a radish mound from which the celery and carrots emanate. Place carrot curls over and around the radish mound and in other nooks and crannies. Keep covered with a slightly damp towel in the refrigerator until ready to serve. Serve with a beverage and a basket of bread.

FRUIT CUPS
Level 2
(1 K-cup = ½ cup)

Fruit cups make a delightful light appetizer for the table. Every variety of fruit and every conceivable combination is fair game for a fruit cup appetizer. For fun, use a halved and hollowed melon or orange as the cup. Garnish the cup with mint or berries.

Some favorite combinations:

- Grapes, orange wedges, and freshly thawed frozen blackberries. Dash of lemon juice over the top.
- Honeydew melon balls, banana slices, and apple slices. Deliciously mellow.
- Pineapple chunks and banana slices served with orange juice over the top.
- Watermelon balls and berries heaped into the center of 1-inch thick rings sliced from honeydew melon or cantaloupe.

TORTILLA CHIPS
Level 3
(1 K-cup = 16 chips)

6 corn tortillas
¼ cup liquid from jar of hot
chili peppers

1 teaspoon paprika
½ teaspoon garlic powder
¼ teaspoon arrowroot

Preheat oven to 500°. Combine chili pepper liquid, paprika, and garlic powder in a saucepan; stir and bring to a boil. Mix arrowroot with 1 teaspoon cold water to make a paste, stir paste into boiling liquid, reduce to simmer, and cook, stirring until liquid thickens. Spread thickened sauce on tortillas, cut each tortilla into eight triangles (pizza pie–style), and place triangles on a wire cake rack. Line cookie sheets with aluminum foil and place cake racks on cookie sheets in oven. Bake 4 or 5 minutes, turn triangles, and bake 4 or 5 minutes more. Serve hot or at room temperature. Makes 48 tortilla chips (about the amount in a medium-sized bag of commercial tortilla chips).

QUICK TORTILLA CHIPS
Level 3
(1 K-cup = 16 chips)

6 corn tortillas
Garlic powder

Onion powder

Preheat oven to 400°. Cut each tortilla into eight triangles. Place triangles on cake rack and bake 6 minutes. Turn chips over, sprinkle with garlic, onion, or both. Bake 3 minutes more. Makes 48 chips (a nice bowlful). Use with any dip. Goes especially well with **Chili Salsa.**

PINEAPPLE BRISTLE
Level 2
(1 K-cup = 7 cubes)

Slice top from pineapple, close to the leaves. Save top. Pare rind from pineapple deep enough so that eyes are removed from pineapple meat. With a long-bladed knife, cut out a cylinder close around the core. Cut the meat to the core in parallel slices about an inch apart all around the pineapple. Hold slices in place with toothpicks fastening them to the core. These slices may all be horizontal, vertical, or diagonal. Now make slices to the core again, but at right angles to the first slices so as to make a grid of 1-inch squares. A toothpick must be placed in each square to keep it fastened to the core. Replace the top of the pineapple. Serve with mace-sprinkled **Sour Cream** or other appropriate dip.

BRUSSELS SPROUTS HORS D'OEUVRE
Level 2
(1 K-cup = 1 cup)

½ cup sliced fresh mushrooms
½ tablespoon garlic juice
¾ cup **Sour Cream**
3 cups small cooked Brussels sprouts

Sauté mushrooms in garlic juice and 1 tablespoon water. Add Brussels sprouts and sour cream and heat. Serve as a hot hors d'oeuvre with toothpicks or little forks. Makes 4 cups.

ZIPPY TOM
Level 2
(1 K-cup = 1 cup)

Hot as you like it, Zippy Tom is a real waker-upper.

1 quart tomato juice
4 lemons
1 teaspoon chili powder
Pepper
Garlic powder
French's Herb Seasoning
4 celery stalk tips, with leaves

Combine tomato juice, the juice of the lemons, and the chili powder. Season to taste with pepper, garlic powder, and herb seasoning. Serve with stalk of celery in each glass. Makes four 8-ounce servings.

FRENCH ONION DIP
Level 3
(1 K-cup = 1 cup)

1 cup **Sour Cream**   2 tablespoons toasted onions

Mix onions with sour cream, cover, and let stand in refrigerator for 24 hours. Delicious! Makes 1 cup.

L.A. BEAN DIP
Level 5
(1 K-cup = 1 cup)

1 cup cooked and drained   2 tablespoons **Yogurt**
   pinto beans   ½ teaspoon onion powder
2 canned California green   Pinch of cayenne pepper
   chilies, chopped

Combine ingredients and mash in small saucepan. Cook to desired consistency. Makes 1¼ cups.

CHEESES, ETC.

SOUR CREAM
Level 2
(1 K-cup = 1 cup)

This recipe makes a *mock* sour cream. No real cream at all is used, yet it is truly delicious. It tastes much like real sour cream, and may be used wherever real sour cream is used. Use it on baked potatoes, in salads, on pancakes, as a dip, etc.

½ gallon skim milk
¼ cup **Buttermilk** *or* commercial cultured buttermilk

Combine ingredients and heat slowly to 95°, stirring constantly. Cover, remove from heat, and let stand in a warm place until coagulated (1 or 2 days). Turn curd into colander lined with 4 layers of cheesecloth. Let drain until whey has drained through (4 to 6 hours). Stir and serve. Makes 2 cups.

CREAM CHEESE `
Level 3
(1 K-cup = ⅔ cup)

2 cups **Sour Cream**

Cut 4 squares of cheesecloth, each large enough to envelop ½ cup of the sour cream. Place ½ cup of sour cream on each cheesecloth square, and bag it up in the cheesecloth, fastening each bag with a wire tie. Place bags on a cake rack over a pan to drain. Let drain 4 to 6 hours or until the consistency of cream cheese is approximated. Makes 1½ cups.

BUTTERMILK
Level 3
(1 K-cup = 1 cup)

It is easy to make buttermilk with a very low fat content. In fact, many commercial buttermilks have fat contents as low as 1-percent fat by *dry weight*. That would put the fat content of the undried product so low, about $1/10$ of 1 percent, as to be totally negligible. Here's the recipe.

1 quart raw skim milk
1 cup **Buttermilk** *or* commercial *cultured* buttermilk*

Warm raw skim milk to 90°, add buttermilk, and stir well. Cover, and let sit in a warm place (80°) 3 to 5 hours. At some point after the first 3 hours of sitting, the buttermilk will be ready. If it *tastes* like buttermilk, it's ready. Pour into a jar and refrigerate. If it sits out for too long after the buttermilk taste has developed, the curd and whey will separate, and the nice uniform buttermilk we want will have been lost. If the buttermilk *does* happen to separate, do not despair. Use it as a fine starter, or simply use it as a "separated" kind of buttermilk. Makes 5 cups of delicious sweet buttermilk.

YOGURT
Level 3
(1 K-cup = 1 cup)

Add a little yogurt to a lot of milk, keep the milk lukewarm (100°) for 10 hours, and like magic you have converted all that milk to yogurt. The easiest way to maintain a constant temperature for the required length of time is with a yogurt maker. Lacking a yogurt maker, try this: heat the milk to 100°, pour it into a warmed thermos bottle, add the yogurt, cap the bottle, wrap it in towels, and place it in a warm,

---

*Use nonfat brands if possible. Otherwise filter out butterfat particles by pouring through several layers of cheesecloth. Realize that repeatedly making **Buttermilk** from already made **Buttermilk** plus skim milk will gradually reduce any initial fat content (created by using a commercial buttermilk) to nearly zero.

draft-free place. Or mix the yogurt and milk, pour into small containers, nestle the containers around a heating pad set at medium, and cover everything up with towels. In any event, here's the recipe:

¼ cup regular nonfat dry milk
1 quart skim milk
3 tablespoons **Yogurt** *or* any commercial yogurt

Combine dry milk with ½ cup of the liquid milk and stir to make a smooth paste. Stir paste into remaining milk. Heat milk to 150°. Heating will kill any unwanted bacteria. As soon as the milk has cooled to 130° you can add the yogurt, which provides the natural bacteria you want. Don't add the yogurt when the temperature is above 135°, though, or you'll kill this bacteria. Maintain at a temperature of 100° for 10 hours, refrigerate, and serve. Makes 1 quart.

SALADS
AND
SALAD DRESSINGS

The caloric-intensity level of a salad depends strongly on the dressing used. In these recipes we have assumed that the dressing plays a small role: to moisten slightly. Caloric intensity may increase if you do more than this.

RAINY DAY SALAD
Level 3
(1 K-cup = 1 cup)

1 large beet, cooked, cooled, and diced

1 large potato, cooked cooled, and diced

1 medium apple, diced

1 medium green pepper, diced

1 stalk celery, diced

Toss all ingredients lightly. Moisten with **Buttermilk Spring Dressing** and tint with some of remaining beet juice. Serves 6.

MACÉDOINE SALAD
Level 3
(1 K-cup = 1 cup)

½ cup vinegar
½ cup water
2 tablespoons lemon juice
1 tablespoon garlic juice
1 cup cooked, diced carrots

2 cups cooked peas
2 cups cooked cauliflower pieces
3 stalks celery, cut into sticks
1 large tomato, sliced

Combine vinegar, water, lemon juice, and garlic juice to make a marinade for the vegetables. Marinate the vegetables separately, 10

169

minutes in the refrigerator. Drain the vegetables, and spoon the carrots and peas into a single pile in the center of a serving platter, alternating a spoonful of carrots with a spoonful of peas. Top the pile with the cauliflower bits. Decorate the serving dish with the celery sticks and tomato slices. Serve cold. Serves 6.

CABBAGE SALAD
Level 2
(1 K-cup = 1 cup)

1 cup chopped cabbage
1 teaspoon green onion tops,
  chopped
¼ cup alfalfa sprouts, firmly
  packed

¼ medium tomato, chopped
¼ cup **Sour Cream**
¼ teaspoon celery seed
⅛ teaspoon paprika
Pepper

Layer cabbage, onion tops, sprouts, and tomato in an individual salad bowl. Combine remaining ingredients and pour over the vegetables. Serves 1.

STUFFED TOMATO SALAD
Level 2
(1 K-cup = 1 cup)

6 medium tomatoes
¼ cup lemon juice
1 teaspoon pepper
2 medium cucumbers,
  peeled and diced finely

1 cup **Sour Cream**
Lettuce

Peel tomatoes, remove and discard a thin slice from the top of each, and remove seeds and some of the pulp. Mix lemon juice and pepper, and pour mixture into one of the tomatoes. Let sit a minute or so, and pour the same mixture into the next tomato. Repeat process for all six tomatoes, then discard lemon and pepper mixture. Invert tomatoes on cake rack, and let drain a few minutes. Fill tomatoes with the diced cucumber mixed with about half the sour cream. Use the remainder of the sour cream to top the tomatoes. Arrange on lettuce leaves, and serve cold. Serves 4.

HOLIDAY SALAD
Level 1
(1 K-cup = 1 cup)

¾ cup fresh asparagus tips,
  steamed
¾ cup fresh green beans,
  steamed
¾ cup diced cucumbers
½ cup raw young peas

½ cup sliced radishes
2 artichoke hearts, cooked
  and sliced
2 egg whites, hard-cooked
  and sliced

Toss all ingredients lightly. Moisten with **Buttermilk Spring Dressing.** Serves 6.

GARDEN GREEN SALAD
Level 1
(1 K-cup = 1 cup)

8 to 12 large leaves of lettuce,
  torn into small pieces
4 onion slices, quartered and
  separated
4 sprigs of parsley, torn up,
  stems removed

¼ cup diced celery
4 Swiss chard leaves, torn
  into small pieces

Toss all ingredients, moisten with favorite dressing, and serve. Serves 4.

ZESTY GREEN SALAD
Level 1
(1 K-cup = 1 cup)

1 cup shredded cabbage
1 cup watercress tops
½ cup raw broccoli flowerets
¼ cup chopped green onion
  tops

½ bunch red lettuce, broken
  into small pieces

Wash, dry, and chill cabbage and watercress. Toss with other ingredients, and moisten with favorite dressing. Serves 6.

INTERNATIONAL SALAD
Level 1
(1 K-cup = 1 cup)

½ pound fresh spinach
1 bunch watercress
1 sweet red onion, thinly sliced

½ small jicama, peeled and thinly sliced
½ cup favorite dressing

Wash spinach and tear into bite-sized pieces. Remove and discard watercress stems, and toss tops with spinach. Make rings from onion slices, and add rings and jicama to salad. Moisten salad with dressing and serve. Serves 4.

PINEAPPLE AND GRAPEFRUIT SALAD
Level 2
(1 K-cup = ⅔ cup)

2 cups crushed pineapple
½ cup grapefruit sections
½ teaspoon mint flakes

2 tablespoons chopped green pepper

Mix all ingredients, chill 1 hour, and serve. Serves 4.

GREEN BEAN ASPIC
Level 2
(1 K-cup = 1 cup)

One 12-ounce can of unsalted vegetable juice
1 tablespoon unflavored gelatin
1 teaspoon lemon juice

1 cup cooked and thoroughly drained French-cut green beans
½ cup cooking liquid from green beans (or water)

Pour ¼ cup vegetable juice into a flat bowl. Sprinkle gelatin evenly over surface, and let soften 5 minutes. Combine lemon juice and beans, toss thoroughly, and set aside. Bring liquid from green beans to a boil, add to gelatin, and stir to completely dissolve all gelatin. Add remaining vegetable juice and stir well. Fold in beans and pour into aspic mold. Chill until set, unmold, and serve. Serves 4.

CARROT AND PEA ASPIC
Level 2
(1 K-cup = 1 cup)

1 tablespoon unflavored
  gelatin
1 cup pure carrot juice
2 tablespoons vinegar
1 tablespoon lemon juice
½ cup clean carrot peelings

1 cup cooked and drained
  peas
1 tablespoon chopped
  pimiento
¼ teaspoon pepper

Sprinkle gelatin over ½ cup water in saucepan, allow 5 minutes to soften, then heat and stir to dissolve gelatin. Stir in all liquid ingredients, followed by remaining ingredients. Pour into serving dish, and chill until set. Serves 4.

TACO SALAD FOR 12
Level 4
(1 K-cup = 1 cup)

1 pound extra-lean ground
  beef, crumbled, cooked,
  drained, and cooled
3 cups grated St. Otto's cheese
One 15-ounce can of kidney
  beans, drained and rinsed
  under cold running water
1 large head lettuce, chopped

2 tomatoes, chopped
1 bunch green onions,
  chopped
1 Recipe of **Quick Tortilla
  Chips**
Dressing: **Chili Salsa** and
  tomato juice, mixed
  to taste

Combine all ingredients except tortilla chips and salsa. Before serving, crush and add tortilla chips. Top with dressing. Serves 12.

TUNA SALAD
Level 1
(1 K-cup = 1 cup)

One 7-ounce can of tuna,
  drained
1 small head lettuce,
  chopped fine
1 cup chopped celery
1 cup diced cucumber
¼ cup vinegar

¼ cup lemon juice
2 teaspoons onion powder
½ teaspoon pepper
4 small tomatoes cut in
  eighths
4 green pepper rings

Mix tuna, lettuce, celery, and cucumber. Mix vinegar, lemon juice, onion powder, and pepper. Combine with tuna mixture. Place mixture on top of tomato wedges. Top with green pepper rings. Serves 4.

TANGY SALAD DRESSING
Level 2
(1 K-cup = 1 cup)

¾ cup tomato juice
3 tablespoons lemon juice
2 tablespoons finely chopped onion
¼ teaspoon pepper

Combine all ingredients, chill, and stir before serving. Makes 1 cup.

BLUE CHEESE DRESSING
Level 3
(1 K-cup = 1 cup)

Overripe blue cheese
1 cup **Sour Cream**

Scrape moldiest areas off blue cheese to get 1 tablespoon of very concentrated blue cheese. Stir into sour cream and thin to desired consistency with **Buttermilk.** Makes 1 cup of delicious blue cheese dressing.

PIMIENTO DRESSING
Level 3
(1 K-cup = 1 cup)

1 cup **Sour Cream**   2 tablespoons sliced pimientos

Place ingredients in blender, chop, then liquify at high speed. A mild, sweet dressing. Makes 1 cup.

GARLIC AND VINEGAR DRESSING
Level 1
(1 K-cup = 1 cup)

2 cloves garlic, sliced   ¼ teaspoon paprika
½ cup vinegar   ½ teaspoon ground thyme
¼ cup water
2 teaspoons frozen apple
  juice concentrate

Combine all ingredients and shake well before serving. Makes ¾ cup.

BUTTERMILK SPRING DRESSING
Level 3
(1 K-cup = 1 cup)

1 cup **Buttermilk**   1 teaspoon onion flakes
1 teaspoon frozen apple juice   1 teaspoon dill weed
  concentrate   Pepper
1 teaspoon lemon juice   Ground allspice

Mix all ingredients except pepper and allspice. Add pepper and ground allspice to taste. (Begin with about ⅛ teaspoon each, and add more if necessary.) Add a little Sap Sago brand cheese for flavor. Chill. Makes 1 cup.

CREAMY SALAD DRESSING
Level 3
(1 K-cup = 1 cup)

1 cup dry-curd cottage cheese
½ cup **Sour Cream**

1 tablespoon lemon juice
½ teaspoon garlic powder

Combine ingredients in blender and blend until smooth. Buttermilk helps the flavor and may be used in thinning. Grated Sap Sago brand cheese adds flavor. Excellent on vegetable or tossed green salads. Makes 1½ cups.

PERFECTION SALAD DRESSING
Level 2
(1 K-cup = ½ cup)

1½ cups unsweetened pineapple juice
1½ cups tomato juice
2 tablespoons fresh lemon juice
2 garlic buds, pressed

2 tablespoons chopped pimiento
2 teaspoons chopped capers
¼ teaspoon freshly ground pepper
¼ teaspoon dry mustard

Combine all ingredients and mix thoroughly. Store tightly covered in refrigerator. Makes 3 cups.

SPICED VINEGAR DRESSING
Level 2
(1 K-cup = 1 cup)

¼ cup wine or cider vinegar
2 tablespoons water
1 tablespoon lemon juice
1 tablespoon onion flakes
1 tablespoon parsley flakes

¼ teaspoon pepper
¼ teaspoon tarragon
¼ teaspoon oregano
¼ teaspoon paprika

Mix ingredients, chill, and stir before serving. Goes great as a light dressing on tossed green salads. Makes ½ cup.

SOUPS
AND
STEWS

CROCK POT SOUP
Level 2
(1 K-cup = 1 cup)

1 large can V-8 juice, unsalted if possible
Fresh vegetables (Whatever you have on hand will work: Cauliflower, broccoli, fresh green beans, potatoes, summer squash, onions, fresh peas, among others)

Wash and cut vegetables into bite-sized pieces. Put all vegetables into a slow cooker. Add the can of V-8 juice and fill the pot to the top with water. Spices may be added, but little is needed. Put slow cooker on high for 2 hours, then turn to low and let cook until vegetables are tender (around 6–8 hours). This is a great soup to put on before going to work in the morning as it will be ready when you get home.

CREAM OF CELERY SOUP
Level 3
(1 K-cup = 1 cup)

2 cups finely chopped celery	2 teaspoons onion powder
2 cups water	1 tablespoon parsley flakes
2 cups **White Sauce**	Dash of nutmeg

Put celery and water into a saucepan, cover, bring to a boil, and simmer until celery is tender (about 10 minutes). Add white sauce and spices, heat through, and serve. Makes 6 cups.

CREAM OF PEA SOUP
Level 3
(1 K-cup = 1 cup)

2 large potatoes
1 cup skim milk
2 cups chopped vegetables:
  celery, onion, green
  pepper

Two 10-ounce packages
  frozen peas
1 teaspoon onion powder
1 teaspoon celery seed
Pepper to taste

Boil potatoes until tender. Peel. Blend until smooth with skim milk. Cook chopped vegetables in 2 cups of water until tender. Add potatoes, peas, spices (and more milk if needed). Heat and serve. Serves 4.

POTATO SOUP
Level 2
(1 K-cup = 1 cup)

1 cup sautéed onions
  (sauté in 2 tablespoons
  water)
2 cups diced potatoes

1 cup chopped celery
1 cup evaporated
  skimmed milk

Add vegetables to 4 cups of boiling water. Cover and boil gently 30 minutes or until vegetables are tender. Add milk. Let simmer 10 minutes. Mash if desired. Serves 8.

GAZPACHO
Level 2
(1 K-cup = 1 cup)

This marvelous cold soup from Spain is simply chopped vegetables in tomato and lime juice. Other liquids may be used in place of tomato juice, and imagination may be used in selecting vegetables. Gazpacho may be used as a soup to go with a salad or as a salad to go with a soup.

2 medium tomatoes
1 green pepper
1 medium zucchini
1 stalk celery
1 clove garlic

1 small red onion
4 cups tomato juice
3 limes
Pepper

Chop all vegetables fine. Purée ⅓ of vegetables with 1 cup of the tomato juice. Combine all ingredients, stir, and chill. Makes about 6 cups.

TOMATO AND ONION SOUP
Level 2
(1 K-cup = 1 cup)

1½ quarts tomato juice
1 medium onion, sliced

1 teaspoon vegetable flakes
3 cloves

Combine all ingredients in a saucepan, bring to a boil, and simmer 5 minutes. Makes 6 cups.

SPLIT PEA SOUP
Level 3
(1 K-cup = 1 cup)

1 pound split peas (2 to 2½ cups)
1 quart **Beef Stock**
1 quart water
½ cup tomato juice

1 cup chopped onions
1 cup chopped celery
¼ teaspoon marjoram
¼ teaspoon pepper
¼ teaspoon thyme

Soak split peas overnight in stock, water, and tomato juice. Drain peas, reserving liquid. Add enough water to liquid to make 2 quarts and return peas to liquid. Bring to boil, reduce heat, and simmer 2 hours. Add vegetables and spices and simmer 30 minutes longer. Bind with arrowroot and serve. Makes 6 cups.

FRENCH ONION SOUP
Level 1
(1 K-cup = 1 cup)

4 medium onions, chopped
4 cups **Beef Stock**

Place ½ cup of onions and 2 tablespoons of stock in a saucepan. Heat slowly until onions start to burn, stirring only occasionally. Stir and continue to brown and even burn onions. Add remaining onions and ¼ cup of stock. Stir, cover, and simmer 5 minutes. Uncover and stir and cook until liquid has evaporated and onions are dry and brown. Add remaining stock and simmer 20 minutes. Makes 5 cups.

GREEK LENTIL SOUP
Level 3
(1 K-cup = 1 cup)

1 cup lentils, washed and
  drained
2 quarts **Chicken Stock,** or
  water
1 medium onion, chopped

1 stalk celery, chopped
1 bay leaf
¼ teaspoon oregano
3 tablespoons tomato paste
2 tablespoons wine vinegar

Without disturbing the boil, slowly pour lentils into vigorously boiling stock. Add all other ingredients except vinegar, reduce heat, and simmer, stirring occasionally, until lentils are very soft (about 1½ hours). Add vinegar. Purée half of the soup in the blender, return puréed portion to pot, mix, heat, and serve. Makes 2 quarts.

BEEF STOCK
Level 1
(1 K-cup = 1 cup)

6 pounds beef bones
1 gallon water
1 onion, cut up
2 carrots, cut up

6 mushrooms, cut up
Other vegetable tops and
  greens, as available
¼ teaspoon pepper

In large pot, bring all ingredients to a boil. Cover and simmer 6 to 10 hours. Strain, chill, and skim fat. Makes about 3 quarts.

CHICKEN STOCK
Level 1
(1 K-cup = 1 cup)

1 whole chicken, disjointed
  (excluding giblets)
½ bay leaf
¼ teaspoon peppercorns
2 stalks celery, whole
1 small onion, quartered

1 bundle fresh herbs
  (parsley, chervil, and thyme)
  tied with string
1 green pepper, seeded and
  quartered

Cut meat from bones and put all ingredients (bones included) into a stew pot with 6 cups of cold water. Gradually bring to a boil, and simmer until meat is tender (2 to 3 hours). Strain, and put aside the chicken meat for use in other recipes. Season with pepper to taste, cool, skim fat, and store in refrigerator or freezer until needed. Makes 1 quart.

QUICK VEGETABLE SOUP
Level 2 or 3 (depending on vegetables)
(1 K-cup = 1 cup)

1 cup leftover cooked
  vegetables

1 cup **Chicken Stock**
½ cup evaporated skim milk

Combine ingredients in blender. Spice as desired and blend. Makes 2½ cups of fabulous cream soup.

MINESTRONE
Level 4
(1 K-cup = 1 cup)

There are many ways to make this old Italian favorite. Rice or pasta may be used in place of the beans, and all kinds of vegetables may be used. Here is our favorite recipe:

1½ cups dried beans (navy, kidney, red, garbanzo, or a mixture)
1 cup fresh green beans
1 small zucchini squash, diced
1 cup shredded spinach or cabbage
1 cup diced tomatoes
½ cup chopped green onions
1 medium onion, chopped
1 cup chopped celery
2 tablespoons parsley flakes
¼ teaspoon savory
½ teaspoon pepper
½ teaspoon thyme
(½ cup dry-curd cottage cheese)

To prepare the dried beans, first clean them, and then either soak them all night in 2 quarts of water or bring them to a boil in 2 quarts of water, simmer 2 minutes, and let stand 1½ hours. Combine the prepared beans, their soaking water, and the fresh green beans in a large soup pot. Bring to a boil, reduce heat, and simmer 45 minutes. Sauté all the remaining vegetables in ¼ cup of water and 1 tablespoon of garlic juice. Add them to the soup pot and continue simmering for another 30 minutes. Add spices and simmer 5 minutes more. If cheese is desired, mix into hot soup and serve. Makes about 2½ quarts.

MINESTRONE WITH RICE
Level 5
(1 K-cup = 1 cup)

½ cup uncooked brown rice
1 medium onion, chopped
1 clove garlic, minced
1 leek, diced
3 stalks celery, chopped
2 medium carrots, diced
2 cups shredded cabbage
2 zucchini, chopped
1½ quarts **Chicken Stock** or water
One 28-ounce can of tomatoes
3 tablespoons tomato paste
2 tablespoons parsley flakes
½ teaspoon thyme
½ teaspoon oregano
3 cups cooked beans (red, navy, lentils, etc.)

Without disturbing the boiling action, slowly add rice to a boiling pot containing all the other ingredients except the beans. Reduce heat and simmer 1 hour. Add beans. Puree ⅓ of the soup in blender, return to pot, stir, heat, and serve. Makes 2 quarts.

MIXED VEGETABLE STEW
Level 2
(1 K-cup = 1 cup)

6 pearl onions, peeled, whole
2½ cups **Chicken Stock**
6 new potatoes, whole, with skins
6 small carrots, cut in half
4 small leeks, chopped
4 small zucchini, chopped
4 stalks celery, chopped
2 medium tomatoes, quartered
1 head cauliflower, broken into flowerets
2 teaspoons arrowroot
2 tablespoons parsley flakes

Boil onions gently in 1 cup water for 20 minutes. Add remaining ingredients except arrowroot and parsley flakes, and simmer until tender (about 1 hour). Add parsley flakes, thicken with arrowroot, and serve. Makes 2½ quarts.

NEW ENGLAND STYLE FISH STEW
Level 3
(1 K-cup = ⅔ cup)

¾ pound black cod or other tender-fleshed fish, cut into 1-inch pieces
3 tablespoons chopped onion
¾ cup vermouth
1½ quarts **Cream of Celery Soup**
¾ teaspoon cayenne pepper

Cook fish and onion in vermouth in Teflon frying pan or saucepan until the odor of the fish is stronger than that of the vermouth. Add cream of celery soup and pepper, and heat to boiling. Simmer a minute or two for thicker soup. Makes 1½ quarts.

BEEF AND GREEN BEAN STEW
Level 4
(1 K-cup = ⅔ cup)

1½ pounds top round, cut
   into ½-inch cubes
1 cup chopped onions

¼ teaspoon pepper
1 cup chopped fresh tomato
2 cups cooked green beans

Brown the meat and onions in a large Teflon frying pan. Add pepper while the mixture is browning. Add ½ cup of water and tomatoes. Cover, and cook over low heat until the meat is tender (about 1 hour). Add the cooked green beans and continue cooking until the beans are heated through. Serves 8.

BEEF STEW
Level 2
(1 K-cup = ⅔ cup)

¾ pound lean stewing beef,
   cut up
3 cloves of fresh garlic,
   sliced
1 onion, coarsely chopped
⅛ teaspoon pepper
3 carrots, coarsely chopped
3 parsnips, coarsely chopped
1 turnip, coarsely chopped
1 potato, coarsely chopped
½ cup fresh mushrooms,
   sliced

1 green pepper, cut
   in chunks
1 onion, sliced
1 medium tomato, peeled, in
   chunks
4 sprigs of parsley, chopped
½ cup dry red wine
2 tablespoons whole wheat
   flour

Trim visible fat from meat and discard. Brown meat over high heat in Teflon frying pan. Bring 1 quart of water to boil and add meat, garlic, onion, and pepper. Return to boil, cover, and simmer 2 hours, stirring occasionally to prevent sticking. Strain to separate meat from broth. Chill broth, skim fat, then recombine meat and broth. Add carrots, parsnips, turnip, and potato, and simmer 15 minutes. Add mushrooms, green pepper, sliced onion, tomato, parsley, and red wine. Simmer 20 more minutes, or until all vegetables are tender. *Prepare brown gravy:* place the 2 tablespoons of whole wheat flour in Teflon frying pan. Heat and stir dry flour with wood spoon, lifting and shaking pan as needed to prevent flour from burning. When flour is medium brown, add ½ cup of broth from stew and stir to thicken. Return thickened gravy to stew, deglazing pan with additional stew broth. Cook and stir stew to thicken. Stew liquid should be light brown and slightly thickened. Serve over rice, noodles, bread, or in bowl by itself. Serves 6 to 8.

MAIN
DISHES

ENCHILADAS
Level 5
(1 K-cup = 1½ enchiladas)

This is a truly excellent vegetarian enchilada dish.

18 corn tortillas

SAUCE:

4 cups tomato sauce
2 to 4 tablespoons **Chili Salsa**

1 tablespoon parsley flakes
1 teaspoon vinegar

FILLING:

4 cups drained **Chili Beans**
  (reserve liquid)
½ cup liquid from **Chili Beans**
One 4-ounce can of chopped
  mushrooms

1 medium onion, chopped
1½ cups dry-curd cottage
  cheese

TOPPING:

1 cup **Sour Cream**

Combine all sauce ingredients and heat through, over low flame. Combine all filling ingredients, except cheese, in saucepan and cook over medium heat 20 minutes. Add the cheese and cook 5 minutes more. In a Teflon pan heat each tortilla on both sides until soft and pliable. Place 2 or 3 tablespoons of filling in the center of each tortilla, roll up, and place in a glass baking dish 11″ × 14″ × 2″. Continue until all filling is used. Pour sauce over enchiladas and top with sour cream. Bake at 350° for 20 minutes. Serves 6.

CHILI BEANS
Level 5
(1 K-cup = 1 cup)

1 pound dried red beans
2 medium onions, chopped
2 stalks celery, chopped
1 medium green pepper,
  chopped

1 teaspoon chili powder
  (more or less, to taste)
½ teaspoon pepper
½ cup **Chili Salsa** (more or
  less, to taste)

Wash and pick over beans. Bring 3 quarts of water to a boil in a 4- to 6-quart saucepan. Add beans a few at a time, so as not to disturb boiling action. Slowly add onions and celery to boiling water. Cook 30 minutes over medium heat. Add green pepper, spices, and **Chili Salsa.** Continue cooking until beans are tender (1 to 1½ hours). Makes 2 quarts. May be frozen for future use.

SPANISH BROWN RICE
Level 5
(1 K-cup = 1 cup)

¾ cup brown rice
¾ cup chopped tomato
¼ cup chopped onion
¼ cup **Chili Salsa**
 2 tablespoons chopped green
  pepper

¼ teaspoon cayenne pepper
⅛ teaspoon paprika
Pinch saffron

In a saucepan, combine all ingredients except rice. Add 2¼ cups water and bring to a boil. Add rice, return to a boil, cover, and simmer 1 hour. Serves 4.

TOSTADAS
Level 5
(1 K-cup = 1 cup of tostadas mashed together)

Refried beans
Corn tortillas
Lettuce

Tomatoes
Onions
Sour Cream

Place tortillas on cookie sheet and place in a preheated 500° oven until crisp. Spread the crisp tortillas with the refried beans and top with lettuce, tomatoes, onions, and **Sour Cream.**

REFRIED BEANS
Level 5
(1 K-cup = 1 cup)

1½ cups dried pinto beans, washed and picked over
1 teaspoon onion powder

2 tablespoons onion flakes
1 teaspoon pepper

Add beans slowly to 1½ quarts boiling water, making sure not to lose the boil. Reduce heat to medium, add spices, cover, and cook just below boiling until beans are tender (about 1½ hours). Drain, mash beans, and stir and cook over medium-to-low flame until beans begin to look dry. Use refried beans in making burritos, tostadas, and other Mexican dishes. Makes 1 quart.

CHILI RELLENOS
Level 3
(1 K-cup = 4" × 3" slice)

Two 7-ounce cans whole California chili peppers
4 or 5 egg whites
2 cups dry-curd cottage cheese
1 red onion, finely chopped

1 tablespoon chopped parsley
1 teaspoon Fines Herbs (Spice Islands mixture of thyme, oregano, marjoram, sage, basil, and rosemary)

Remove and discard seeds and wash each chili. Mix cheese with all ingredients except chilies. Layer half the chilies on the bottom of a small (8" × 8" × 2") casserole dish. Spread the cheese mixture over the chilies. Layer the rest of chilies on top. Top with **Chili Salsa.** Bake 30 minutes at 350°. Serves 6 to 8.

ZUCCHINI LASAGNA
Level 4
(1 K-cup = 3" × 4" slice, 1" thick)

4 small zucchini squash,
  peeled and sliced
  lengthwise
2 cups grated St. Otto's cheese
2 cups dry-curd cottage
  cheese
1 cup egg whites (about 8
  eggs)

¼ cup parsley flakes
½ teaspoon pepper
1 pound lasagna noodles,
  cooked *al dente* and
  drained
1 quart **Spaghetti Sauce**

Cook zucchini 10 minutes in vegetable steamer. Make a cheese mixture by combining cheese with egg whites, parsley, and pepper. Layer ingredients as follows: noodles, cheese mixture, spaghetti sauce, zucchini, cheese mixture, spaghetti sauce. Repeat until all ingredients have been used. Bake 1 hour at 350°. Serves 8.

SPINACH LASAGNA
Level 4
(1 K-cup = 3" × 4" slice, 1" thick)

Wow! Who would think spinach would go so well in a lasagna dish! Try this recipe for a real taste treat.

2 bunches fresh spinach
1 pound lasagna noodles
2 small onions, chopped
½ cup sliced mushrooms
½ large green pepper,
  chopped
½ teaspoon minced garlic
One 28-ounce can of tomatoes,
  with half the liquid in the
  can

1 teaspoon oregano flakes
1 teaspoon basil flakes
2½ cups dry-curd cottage
  cheese
2 egg whites
1 cup grated St. Otto's cheese
1 tablespoon parsley flakes
½ teaspoon pepper
Bread crumbs

Prepare spinach: wash leaves thoroughly and remove stems; wilt spinach by placing in colander and then plunging in hot water 10 seconds; chop wilted spinach fine. *Prepare noodles:* cook and drain. *Prepare sauce:* sauté onions, mushrooms, green pepper, and garlic in 3 tablespoons water; add the canned tomatoes and juice after chopping 2 or 3 seconds in blender; add spices; simmer 30 minutes; then add spinach. *Prepare cheese mixture:* mix cottage cheese with egg whites, then add fresh cheese, parsley flakes, and pepper. *Prepare lasagna for baking:* place one third of the noodles in the bottom of a baking dish 13″ × 9″ × 2″; layer in one third of cheese mixture followed by one third of sauce; repeat process twice more, using up all of the noodles, cheese mixture, and sauce. Top with bread crumbs and bake at 350° for about 30 minutes. Serves 10.

MANICOTTI
Level 4
(1 K-cup = 2 manicottis)

12 manicotti noodles (usually the contents of a single package)

2 cups dry-curd cottage cheese

1 cup grated St. Otto's cheese

3 egg whites

2 teaspoons parsley flakes

½ teaspoon pepper

(½ teaspoon thyme)

(½ teaspoon basil)

(½ teaspoon garlic powder)

1 quart **Spaghetti Sauce**

Cook manicotti noodles to *al dente* stage. Drain and place in cool water while casserole is being made. Combine cottage cheese, fresh cheese, egg whites, and spices, adding a little water if necessary to optimize the mixture for stuffing. Spread a cup of the spaghetti sauce over the bottom of a baking dish. One by one, drain each noodle, stuff it with the cottage cheese mixture, using a long-handled spoon, and lay it in the baking dish. Pour remaining sauce over top and bake at 375° until slightly browned on top (about 30 minutes). Serves 6.

NADA'S VEGETARIAN CABBAGE ROLLS
Level 3
(1 K-cup = 3 cabbage rolls)

1 large head cabbage

STUFFING:

2 cups cooked and drained red, kidney, or garbanzo beans
1 cup chopped onion
1 cup diced celery
½ cup partially cooked brown rice (to partially cook, boil
   vigorously 10 minutes in 1½ cups water; drain)
One 16-ounce can of whole tomatoes, drained and chopped finely
1 cup tomato sauce
1 egg white
1 tablespoon parsley flakes
½ teaspoon garlic flakes
¼ teaspoon oregano flakes
⅛ teaspoon pepper

SAUCE:

One 28-ounce can of tomatoes packed in puree (blended 5 seconds
   in blender)
1 stalk celery, diced
1 tablespoon parsley flakes
⅛ teaspoon garlic flakes

Place whole cabbage in a large pot, add 1 cup water, cover tightly,
and steam until cabbage leaves can be separated (about 20 minutes).
Mix all stuffing ingredients together. On each cabbage leaf, place a
small amount of stuffing (about 3 tablespoons), tuck in ends, roll up,
and place in shallow baking dish. Largest leaves may be cut in half to
keep rolls more or less uniform in size. Combine sauce ingredients.
Chop unused center of cabbage, and add ½ cup of this chopped
cabbage to sauce. Pour sauce over cabbage rolls, cover, and bake 25
minutes at 350°. Remove cover and bake 20 minutes more. Makes
about 16 rolls. Serves 8.

FALAFELS
Level 3
(1 K-cup = 1 falafel)

4 cups cooked garbanzos
4 egg whites
1 cup finely chopped onions
2 teaspoons chopped
  parsley
½ teaspoon garlic powder

½ teaspoon basil
Pepper
¾ cup matzo meal
  (Manischewitz unsalted)
¼ cup potato pancake mix
  (Manischewitz)

Put garbanzos and a small amount of the cooking liquid in the blender. Blend until smooth. Mix the garbanzos, egg whites, onions, and spices in a large bowl. Add sufficient matzo meal and pancake mix to make stiff enough to form small balls (about 1 inch). Bake on Teflon pan at 350° for 15–20 minutes. *Serve in pita bread:* 3 to 4 balls to half a pita. Top with lettuce, tomato, onions, and a *very* small amount of dill pickles. If desired, top with **Buttermilk Spring Dressing** or a mixture of tomato sauce and a small bit of prepared mustard. **Gazpacho** also makes a great topping.

PIZZA
Level 5
(1 K-cup = 6″ × 4″ slice, ½″ thick)

DOUGH:
3½ cups flour (half whole wheat and half white flour)
  1 package yeast dissolved in ⅓ cup warm water
1¼ cups tepid water

Mix and knead. Let rise 3 to 4 hours then punch down. Flatten dough on Teflon baking pan and let rise again (about 1 hour).

TOPPING:
3 cups **Spaghetti Sauce**
1 cup chopped onions
1 cup chopped green
  peppers

1 cup sliced fresh mushrooms
1 cup dry-curd cottage
  cheese
(Sap Sago cheese, grated)

After dough has risen ½ hour the second time, spread sauce on top and let dough rise the last ½ hour. Top with vegetables, then with cheeses. Bake 25 minutes at 375°. Makes one large pizza.

MUSHROOM AND POTATO GARDEN
Level 3
(1 K-cup = ½ serving)

4 large potatoes, suitable for baking
1½ cups **Sour Cream**
½ pound fresh mushrooms, sliced
1 tablespoon garlic juice
1 teaspoon onion juice
1½ cups alfalfa sprouts
3 medium tomatoes, cut into wedges
1 green pepper, sliced

Wash potatoes and bake until done at 350° (about 1 hour). Sauté mushrooms in garlic juice, onion juice, and 2 tablespoons water, until liquid is gone. Place each potato in center of individual serving plate, slit open, fill with sour cream, and top with mushrooms. Surround each potato with heaps of sprouts. Symmetrically arrange tomato wedges and pepper slices around the potato, on top of the sprouts. Beautiful and delicious! Each potato arrangement is one serving. Serves 4.

VEGETABLE CASSEROLE
Level 4
(1 K-cup = 1 cup)

Use those aging vegetables in the vegetable bin and the leftover vegetables from Tuesday night's dinner in this delicious, quick casserole. This recipe is a "for instance." Use it as a guide, but use whatever's on hand. (The onions and the tomatoes are always used.) Hard fresh vegetables, like carrots, will need to be partially cooked first.

4 cups cooked and drained
    shell or elbow macaroni
2 large tomatoes, sliced
1 large onion, sliced
1 medium zucchini, sliced

1 cup sliced fresh mushrooms
1 cup fresh broccoli pieces
1 cup grated St. Otto's cheese
2 cups **Versatility Sauce**

In a glass baking dish 13" × 9" × 2", layer the ingredients in the following sequence:
    half the onions and tomatoes;
    a third of the macaroni;
    half the zucchini, mushrooms, broccoli, and cheese;
    another third of the macaroni;
    remainder of zucchini, mushrooms, broccoli, and cheese;
    remainder of the macaroni.
    Pour sauce over casserole. Add remainder of onions and tomatoes as a topping layer. Cover and bake 30 minutes at 350°. Serves 6.

SUMMER GARDEN PLATE
Level 1
(1 K-cup = ½ serving)

4 ears fresh corn, shucked
    and cleaned
4 small summer squash
    (cymling), sliced
2 medium zucchini, sliced

2 medium crookneck squash,
    sliced
⅓ medium red onion,
    sliced thin
½ cup **Sour Cream**

Bring 2 quarts of water to a boil, drop in ears of corn, and boil until tender (about 10 minutes). Steam squash in a covered frying pan, using 2 or 3 tablespoons water and a hot flame. The squash will require only 2 or 3 minutes of steaming. It should not be overcooked so as to brown, nor oversteamed so as to become soggy. Avoid crowding the squash in the frying pan. Cook about a cup of the squash slices at a time, keeping the already-cooked squash warm while subsequent batches are being cooked. Serve squash and corn piping hot on individual serving plates. Garnish each plate with the onion slices. Use the sour cream in place of butter on the corn. (Delicious!) A sourdough bread and a cool beverage go well with this dish. Makes 4 servings.

MOM'S SPICY EGGPLANT
Level 2
(1 K-cup = 1 cup)

1 medium eggplant sliced, unpeeled, into ¼-inch slices
One 15-ounce can of green beans, drained
1 large onion, sliced thin
2 tablespoons diced canned California green chilies
One 15-ounce can of whole tomatoes, cut up
(2 ounces raw hamburger, broken into small pieces)
¼ teaspoon thyme

Combine ingredients in a medium baking dish, cover securely, and bake 1 hour at 350°. Serves 4.

GREEN BEAN CASSEROLE
Level 2
(1 K-cup = 1 cup)

1½ pounds fresh green beans
¼ teaspoon pepper
1 tablespoon **Chili Salsa** (or more, to taste)

½ cups grated St. Otto's cheese
2 cups **Versatility Sauce**
1 cup dry-curd cottage cheese

TOPPINGS:
(½ cup grated St. Otto's cheese)
(¼ cup fresh bread crumbs)
(3 hard-cooked egg whites, shredded)

Simmer green beans, covered, in ½ cup water for 20 minutes. Drain. Combine green beans, pepper, **Chili Salsa,** and cheese in shallow glass baking dish. Pour sauce over all, top with any or all of toppings, and bake at 350° until surface browns (about 20 minutes). Serves 6.

SWEET AND SOUR VEGETABLES
Level 2
(1 K-cup = 1 cup)

1 tablespoon cornstarch
2 tablespoons vermouth
¾ cup **Chicken Stock** *or* water
One 8-ounce can of crushed
  pineapple, juice-packed
½ cup bean sprouts
¼ cup alfalfa sprouts
 2 tablespoons sliced green
  onions, tops and bottoms
 2 small carrots, cut in thin,
  2-inch-long strips
½ cup thinly sliced Chinese
  celery-cabbage
½ teaspoon grated fresh
  ginger root (or ¼ teaspoon
  ground ginger)
½ cup sliced fresh mushrooms

¼ cup jicama, cut in strips
  ½" × 2" × ⅛"
  or substitute canned
  water chestnuts
10 snow pea pods
¼ cup green pepper, in
  ¾-inch pieces
¼ cup fresh broccoli stems,
  cut across grain in thin
  slices
 1 Jerusalem artichoke, sliced
  thin
 2 tablespoons chopped
  pimiento
 1 tablespoon vinegar
(½ pound cooked chicken, in
  small cubes)

Mix cornstarch and vermouth. Combine with chicken stock and juice from pineapple, in 2-quart saucepan, and cover over medium heat, stirring constantly, until thickened. Add remaining ingredients, and simmer, stirring frequently, until vegetables are just slightly tender but still crisp and colorful (6 to 7 minutes). Serve over cooked brown rice. Serves 4.

TEFLON-FRIED ZUCCHINI
Level 1
(1 K-cup = 1 cup)

So fast and so good, this dish is perfect for a fast lunch or a last-minute side dish at dinner.

4 medium zucchini, sliced   Pepper
2 tablespoons garlic juice

Put half (about 1 cup) of the zucchini into a frying pan with 1 tablespoon of the liquid garlic, 2 tablespoons of water, and a dash of pepper. Cover tightly, and cook 2 or 3 minutes over a hot flame, occasionally shaking the pan to stir. Repeat process for the other half of the zucchini. Serve immediately. Fantastic! Serves 4.

CAULIFLOWER IN BLOOM
Level 1
(1 K-cup = 1 serving)

1 head cauliflower	Thyme
2 bunches broccoli	Savory
2 lemons, cut in length- wise wedges	

Cut out green stem and pulpy center of cauliflower. Rinse. Cut off the inedible bottom parts of the broccoli stems, and wash broccoli. Place a vegetable steaming rack at bottom of a large pot, and add water just to the level of the rack bottom. Place cauliflower and broccoli in rack, add spices to taste, cover pot tightly, and steam until tender (about 20 minutes). Serve on a large platter with cauliflower in center and broccoli groups radiating outward, interspersed with lemon wedges. Makes 6 servings.

GARDEN CASSEROLE
Level 3
(1 K-cup = 1 cup)

1 medium onion, chopped	2 large zucchini, sliced
1 teaspoon chili powder	1 cup corn kernels,
1 teaspoon oregano	preferably fresh off the cob
⅛ tablespoon ground cumin	2 medium tomatoes, sliced
Dash of cayenne pepper	½ cup tiny sourdough bread
1 medium green pepper, cut	cubes
in strips	Paprika

Place onions, spices, and ¾ cup water in small saucepan, and heat to boiling. Pour into casserole dish; add peppers, zucchini, and corn;

cover; and bake 1 hour at 350°. Then stir in tomatoes, top with bread cubes, sprinkle with a bit of paprika, and bake uncovered an additional 25 minutes. Serves 4.

CHICKEN BREAST PAPRIKA
Level 3
(1 K-cup = ⅔ cup)

¾ pound of chicken breasts
½ cup **Buttermilk**
1 teaspoon paprika
1 cup flat or crinkly noodles
2 cups sliced mushrooms
¼ cup chopped onion

¼ cup chopped celery
2 tablespoons chopped green pepper
½ cup vermouth
2 cups **Sour Cream**
Chopped chives for garnish

Preheat oven to 450°. Remove skin and fat from chicken breasts. Cut the meat from the bones, into filets. Marinate 2 hours in buttermilk and paprika. Arrange in a single layer in a flat baking dish, smothered in marinade. (If desired, top with freshly ground pepper.) Bake 20 minutes. While chicken is baking, cook noodles. Meanwhile sauté vegetables in vermouth, in a covered pan. Boil off excess liquid. Add sour cream and heat gently until warm. Add the cooking juices from the chicken (which by now should be done) and mix. Serve chicken on bed of noodles topped with vegetable–sour cream mixture. Garnish with chopped chives. Serves 4.

ARROZ CON POLLO
(Rice with chicken)
Level 5
(1 K-cup = 1 chicken breast)

4 chicken breasts, skinned and trimmed of visible fat
¼ cup vermouth
1 cup brown rice
1 cup sliced fresh mushrooms
1 cup chopped onion
2 cloves garlic, sliced

2½ cups **Chicken Stock**
One 28-ounce can of whole tomatoes
¼ cup chopped pimiento
2 tablespoons chopped fresh parsley
½ teaspoon pepper
Pinch of saffron

Moisten chicken with vermouth, and brown in broiler, 3 inches from element. With pastry brush baste frequently to prevent dryness, using cooking juices and water (or chicken broth). Remove chicken when lightly browned, and arrange in casserole dish. In separate pan, combine rice, mushrooms, onions, and garlic in ¼ cup stock and cook over moderate heat for 5 minutes. Add remaining stock, bring to a boil, cover, and simmer 20 minutes at very low heat. Add remaining ingredients, heat to boiling, and pour over chicken in casserole. Cover and bake at 350° for 50 minutes. Remove cover and cook 10 minutes more. Serves 4.

CHICKEN-LACED MANICOTTI
Level 4
(1 K-cup = 1 serving)

¾ pound of chicken breast
4 manicotti shells, cooked
  al dente and cooled
1½ cups **Chicken Stuffing**

¼ pound St. Otto's cheese,
  cut into very thin slices
3 sprigs of fresh rosemary
2¼ cups **Mushroom Sauce**

Remove skin, bones, and fat from chicken, being careful to preserve the chicken meat in pieces that are as large as possible. Cut chicken into long strips 1 inch wide. Carefully fill manicotti shells with stuffing, and place stuffed shells in shallow baking dish, leaving ample space between. Wrap chicken strips diagonally around manicotti shells (about 2 strips per shell). Arrange cheese slices on top of manicotti shells, in between chicken strips. Place rosemary needles between manicotti shells, and pour sauce over all. Preheat oven to broil temperature. Insert casserole, and immediately reduce oven setting to 350°. Bake 30 minutes and serve. Serves 4.

CHICKEN STUFFING
Level 5
(1 K-cup = 1 cup)

½ cup wild rice, rinsed
1 tablespoon regular nonfat
  dry milk
1 tablespoon parsley flakes

3 egg whites
⅛ teaspoon pepper
¾ cup dry-curd cottage
  cheese

Place rice in small saucepan, add 2 cups water, cover, and simmer 35 minutes. Drain rice thoroughly. Combine dry milk, parsley flakes, egg whites, and pepper, crushing lumps of milk to make smooth. Stir in cheese and rice. Makes 1½ cups.

JUICY VEGETABLED CHICKEN
Level 3
(1 K-cup = ½ serving)

4 small chicken breasts (combined weight less than 1 pound)
2 cloves garlic, sliced
3 medium green peppers, sliced
2 cups thin onion slices
½ cup **Chicken Stock**
½ cup dry sherry wine
1 bay leaf
¼ teaspoon pepper
1 pound fresh mushrooms, sliced
2 medium tomatoes, cut in wedges
2 tablespoons cornstarch
¼ cup chopped fresh parsley
2 tablespoons chopped pimiento

Remove skin and fat from chicken and brown under the broiler. Place garlic slices in large skillet with 2 tablespoons water and cook over high heat for 2 minutes. Add browned chicken, green peppers, onion, stock, wine, bay leaf, and pepper. Cover, and cook 20 minutes over low heat, stirring occasionally. Add mushrooms and tomatoes and cook 10 minutes more. Remove bay leaf. Stir in a mixture of the cornstarch combined with 2 tablespoons of water, and cook and stir occasionally until thickened. Sprinkle with parsley and pimiento and serve. Serves 4.

YANKEE CHICKEN GUMBO
Level 3
(1 K-cup = ⅔ cup)

One 8-ounce can of tomatoes
1½ cups **Chicken Stock**
  1 small zucchini, sliced
  1 medium onion, chopped
  1 green pepper, chopped
  1 clove garlic, finely
    chopped
  1 teaspoon paprika
Pinch of saffron

½ teaspoon thyme
¼ teaspoon pepper
⅛ teaspoon cayenne pepper
 1 chicken breast (½ pound)
 5 fresh okra
 1 potato
¼ cup freshly chopped
  parsley
 2 teaspoons cornstarch

Combine tomatoes, stock, zucchini, onion, green pepper, garlic, and spices in a large pot. Bring to a boil, cover, and simmer for 10 minutes. Remove fat and bones from chicken breast, cut meat into ½-inch cubes, and Teflon-fry until white and separate. Cut okra into ½-inch slices. Cut peeled potato into ½-inch cubes. Add chicken, okra, potato, and parsley to simmering pot, and cook until all vegetables are tender. Mix cornstarch with small amount of water, add to pot, and cook, stirring constantly, until thickened, boiling down to reduce liquid if necessary. Serve over brown rice. Serves 4.

NEPTUNE'S CHOWDER
Level 3
(1 K-cup = ⅔ cup)

2 pounds fillets of firm-fleshed
  fish (e.g., halibut, red
  snapper, sea bass, or
  scallops)
3 large potatoes
1 medium onion, chopped
1 medium leek, chopped
1 stalk celery, chopped
1 clove garlic, minced finely
1 large carrot, diced

One 28-ounce can of tomatoes,
  chopped
 1 cup tomato sauce
 2 tablespoons parsley flakes
 2 bay leaves
¾ teaspoon thyme
Dash of pepper
¾ cup sherry wine
 1 medium lemon
 3 tablespoons cornstarch

Cut fish into 1½-inch cubes and set aside. Boil potatoes until tender but not soft, then peel and dice. Place onion, leek, celery, and garlic in a large soup pot. Add ½ cup water, cover, and cook over medium heat until vegetables are tender and slightly yellow (about 15 minutes). Add carrot, tomatoes, tomato sauce, and spices, and simmer, covered, 30 minutes. Add wine, juice of the lemon, the cut-up fish, and the diced potatoes, and simmer 20 minutes more. Mix cornstarch with ⅓ cup cold water, stir into the simmering pot, and cook and stir until chowder thickens. Cook a few minutes more and serve. Serves 8.

BRINY DEEP SALMON LOAF
Level 4
(1 K-cup = ⅔ cup)

One 7¾-ounce can of salmon, drained
3 cups soft bread crumbs
3 egg whites
½ cup skim milk
½ cup chopped onion
2 tablespoons parsley flakes
½ teaspoon tarragon
2½ cups **Curried Pea Sauce**

Combine all ingredients except pea sauce, mixing and mashing well to distribute salmon, seasonings, and wet ingredients thoroughly in bread crumbs. Shape mixture in a 8″ × 8″ × 2″ Teflon pan. Bake 25 minutes at 400°. Pour hot curried pea sauce over entire surface of salmon loaf, and serve. Serves 4.

BROILED FISH FILLETS
Level 3
(1 K-cup = 4 ounces)

1 pound tender-fleshed fish fillets (such as cod, whiting, or flounder)
2 medium lemons
¼ teaspoon basil
⅛ teaspoon thyme
⅛ teaspoon pepper
¼ cup dry white wine
Fresh parsley sprigs

In a shallow pan, arrange fillets in a single layer. Brush or sprinkle fish with juice from one of the lemons, then sprinkle with basil, thyme, and pepper. Pour wine into pan around (not on top of) fish. Broil close to heat until fish begins to brown and looks slightly dry, with juices congealing. Do not attempt to turn fish. Serve with parsley trim and wedges cut from remaining lemon. Serves 6.

BEEFARONI
Level 4
(1 K-cup = ⅔ cup)

1 cup elbow macaroni
2 cups **Spahgetti Sauce**
½ pound leanest ground beef, broken in pieces

1½ cups **Sour Cream**
½ cup grated St. Otto's cheese
½ cup bread crumbs

Cook macaroni. Combine macaroni, spaghetti sauce, and ground beef in baking dish. Spread top with sour cream. Sprinkle with fresh cheese and bread crumbs. Bake at 400° for 20 minutes. Serves 4.

NADA'S BEEF CABBAGE ROLLS
Level 3
(1 K-cup = 2 cabbage rolls)

A simple substitution in **Nada's Vegetarian Cabbage Rolls** makes the dish into a delicious, meaty-flavored beef dish. In place of the called-for 2 cups of beans, substitute ½ pound of leanest ground beef mixed with 1½ cups cooked garbanzo beans. Otherwise, follow the directions exactly. Serves 8.

TIP KABOBS
Level 4
(1 K-cup = 3 skewers, 1 meat cube per skewer)

Tip Kabobs offer a real change of pace for dinnertime. Family and friends can make and cook their own and enjoy being together while they cook. Small children love them, and will ask again and again for another tip kabob dinner. They're terrific at dinner parties, offering guests an ideal opportunity to talk and get acquainted as they prepare and cook their own. Best of all, tip kabob ingredients can be made up in advance and simply set out at dinnertime. Use 1 pound of meat for each 6 people and marinate the meat in either marinade (not both) as instructed below. Skewer meat and other skewering ingredients, closely packed, on bamboo skewers that have been soaked 24 hours in water to prevent their burning. Broil on broiling rack or over hibachi.

MEAT:
Lean sirloin tip steak, cut into 1-inch cubes

WINE AND GARLIC MARINADE:
Use these amounts for each pound of meat, and marinate meat 3 to 6 hours.

2 cups dry white wine	2 cloves garlic, chopped fine
¼ cup vinegar (preferably champagne vinegar)	1 teaspoon garlic powder
	2 teaspoons onion powder
2 teaspoons lemon juice	¼ teaspoon pepper

VEGETABLE MARINADE:
Use these amounts for each pound of meat, and marinate meat 24 hours in refrigerator.

2 tablespoons lemon juice	2 teaspoons parsley flakes
1 cup vegetable juice	½ teaspoon whole celery seed
¼ cup cider vinegar	¼ teaspoon pepper
2 tablespoons vegetable flakes	

SKEWERING INGREDIENTS:
Place these items (or other tasty substitutions) in separate bowls, for skewering.

Peeled and parboiled boiling
onions
Green peppers cut in 1-inch
squares
Cherry tomatoes
Fresh mushroom caps

Eggplant cut in 1-inch cubes
and marinated in vegetable
marinade above
Chunks of fresh pineapple
And, of course, marinated
meat cubes

CHILI CON CARNE
Level 5
(1 K-cup = 1 cup)

1 cup dried kidney or
pinto beans
½ pound leanest ground beef
1 large onion, sliced
1 green pepper, coarsely
chopped

One 15-ounce can tomatoes
2 tablespoons chili powder
1 bay leaf
¼ teaspoon cumin
½ teaspoon oregano

Rinse beans. Bring beans to a boil in 3 cups of water, simmer 3 minutes, and let stand 1 hour. Cook until tender (2 to 3 hours). Drain beans, reserving liquid. Brown meat in large Teflon pan. Discard all fat. Add remaining ingredients to meat, stirring and cooking over high heat until mixture boils. Add drained beans to mixture, cover, and simmer at very low temperature for 1 to 1½ hours, stirring occasionally to prevent sticking. Add bean liquid if mixture becomes too thick. Remove bay leaf. Serves 4 to 6.

The next three recipes, while not really main dishes, make excellent accompaniments to main dishes.

CARROTS WITH PINEAPPLE
Level 2
(1 K-cup = ½ cup)

Neither carrots nor pineapple ever tasted so good. This sweet and delicious recipe comes from a Hindu ashram in Boston. Use it as a side dish when serving pastas, bean dishes, or meat dishes.

4 medium carrots, peeled and diagonally sliced (¼-inch slices)
One 28-ounce can of juice-packed crushed pineapple
   (room temperature)
⅛ teaspoon ginger

Place carrots in saucepan and add juice from canned pineapple. (Add additional pineapple juice or water, if necessary, to cover carrots.) Cover, boil gently until carrots are tender (about 20 minutes), and drain. Stir in crushed pineapple and ginger. Serves 4.

MIXED GREENS
Level 1
(1 K-cup = 1 cup)

½ pound spinach, washed
   and chopped
½ pound swiss chard,
   washed and chopped

3 sprigs parsley, chopped
2 large green onion
   bottoms, chopped
¼ teaspoon Italian Seasoning

Combine still-wet vegetables and seasoning in pot. Adding no water, cover tightly, and cook 5 to 10 minutes over low heat. Serve hot. Serves 4.

STOVE POTATOES
Level 3
(1 K-cup = 1 cup)

5 medium potatoes, peeled
   and diced
1 large onion, diced

1 tablespoon parsley flakes
½ teaspoon pepper

Combine all ingredients in saucepan, add enough water to cover, and cook over medium flame until tender (about 20 minutes). Drain and serve. So good and so easy to fix! Serves 4.

SAUCES

VERSATILITY SAUCE
Level 3
(1 K-cup = 1 cup)

This delicious sauce can really "make" a dish. Use it on **Green Bean Casserole** or over any pasta. Goes well on meats and other dishes too.

1 medium green pepper, chopped fine
1 medium onion, chopped fine
1 stalk celery, diced
1 clove garlic, minced

2 tablespoons whole wheat flour
1½ cups tomato juice
½ teaspoon oregano flakes
½ teaspoon basil

Sauté green pepper, onion, celery, and garlic in 2 tablespoons water, until tender (about 5 minutes). Sprinkle flour evenly over top, add tomato juice, oregano, and basil, and cook and stir over medium heat until sauce thickens. Makes 2 cups.

CURRIED PEA SAUCE
Level 4
(1 K-cup = 1 cup)

One 10-ounce package of frozen peas
1 cup skim milk
2 tablespoons chopped pimiento

1 tablespoon cornstarch
1 teaspoon curry powder

Place peas in saucepan, add ½ cup water, cover, and cook over medium heat until tender (5 to 8 minutes). Add milk and pimiento, and heat to just below boiling. Make paste of cornstarch, curry powder, and 2 tablespoons of water. Stir into peas and cook over low heat until thickened. Makes 2½ cups. Serve with **Briny Deep Salmon Loaf** or any other fish or chicken entrée needing a sauce.

COMPROMISE WHITE SAUCE
Level 5
(1 K-cup = 1 cup)

This white sauce is a compromise. It contains a tablespoon of butter. We have included it because, while it does contain fat (butter is nearly 100 percent fat), it matches in taste and texture the white sauces that are commonly used. However, 1 cup of this white sauce carries with it over 130 calories in fat. One would be well advised not to consume more than ½ cup daily.

1 tablespoon butter	2 tablespoons flour
1 cup skim milk	Dash of white pepper

Combine butter and 1 tablespoon of the skim milk in a small sauce-pan. Heat and mix until butter melts and is evenly mixed with milk. Remove from heat, add flour, and mix. Begin cooking over low heat. Add small amounts of the remaining milk while cooking and stirring constantly. Use all milk. Cook slowly until thickening is nearly complete. Add pepper and cook until fully thickened. Makes 1 cup.

MUSHROOM SAUCE
Level 4
(1 K-cup = 1 cup)

Simple as can be, this sauce is terrific as a base for tuna and other casseroles.

½ cup sliced fresh mushrooms	2 tablespoons water
1 tablespoon garlic juice	2 cups **White Sauce**

Sauté mushrooms in garlic juice and water. Combine with white sauce and heat. Makes 2¼ cups.

TUNA MUSHROOM SAUCE
Level 5
(1 K-cup = 1 cup)

½ cup sliced fresh mushrooms
1 tablespoon vermouth
One 7-ounce can of tuna,
   undrained

1 cup **White Sauce**
½ teaspoon powdered
   mushroom
White pepper

Sauté mushrooms in vermouth and 1 tablespoon water. Combine all ingredients in saucepan and cook and stir to blend and thicken. Makes 2 cups.

SPAGHETTI SAUCE
Level 2
(1 K-cup = 1 cup)

Two 28-ounce cans of tomatoes
2 cups tomato sauce
1 large onion, chopped
½ cup dry burgundy wine
1 tablespoon grated green
   cheese

1½ tablespoons oregano flakes
1 teaspoon garlic powder
1 teaspoon basil

Blend tomatoes in blender, place in a saucepan, and cook and stir over high flame until cooked down to a thick consistency (about 45 minutes). Prepare and add remaining ingredients while tomatoes are cooking. Makes 2½ quarts.

SPAGHETTI SAUCE #6
Level 2
(1 K-cup = 1 cup)

This recipe, straight from the *Live Longer Now Cookbook,* is a favorite at the Institute of Health.

Three 28-ounce cans of
tomatoes, packed in purée
2 cups chopped fresh
mushrooms
2 medium onions, chopped
1 medium green pepper,
chopped

1 stalk celery, chopped
1 tablespoon garlic flakes
1 tablespoon parsley flakes
1 tablespoon oregano flakes
1 teaspoon pepper
1 teaspoon basil
1 teaspoon dried thyme leaves

Chop tomatoes briefly in blender. Combine all ingredients in a large saucepan, add ¼ cup water, cover, and simmer slowly 2 hours. Makes 3 quarts.

CHILI SALSA
Level 3
(1 K-cup = 1 cup)

3 fresh jalapeño chilies
3 fresh yellow chilies
2 fresh California green
chilies
2 medium tomatoes,
chopped
(4 tomatillos)

½ medium onion, chopped
1 stalk celery, chopped fine
1 tablespoon vinegar
½ teaspoon coriander seeds
(or ¼ cup finely chopped
cilantro)
½ teaspoon garlic flakes

Seed the chilies, saving a teaspoon or so of the seeds to make the salsa hot. Chop the chilies, and combine all ingredients except the seeds in a saucepan. Add ½ cup water. Add seeds ⅛ teaspoon at a time, tasting for hotness at each addition. Stop at desired hotness. Cover and simmer 3 hours. Use on tacos, in beans, on refried beans, in burritos, or in any other dish to give a spicy Mexican flavor. Store in refrigerator or freezer. Makes 2 cups.

VEGETABLE POWDER
Level 1

½ cup vegetable flakes   1 tablespoon onion flakes
1 tablespoon parsley flakes   ¼ teaspoon chervil

Pulverize all ingredients in blender. Store in airtight jar until needed. Use to enrich soups, stews, meats, and cooked vegetables. Makes ¼ cup.

BREADS

LEAN LONGEVITY BREAD
Level 3
(1 K-cup = 1 slice)

The honey and salt in this recipe are necessary for proper rising of the dough. They don't affect the taste of the bread, but they greatly affect the action of the dough. The quantities used are small enough to be of no health consequence.

4½ cups whole wheat flour	1 tablespoon dry yeast
½ teaspoon salt	½ teaspoon honey

Put 2 cups of water in a saucepan and heat to lukewarm. Remove from heat and add the dry yeast and honey. Cover and let sit 15 minutes. Combine with flour and salt in a large bowl and knead for 10 minutes. Set bowl in a sink filled with hot water, cover with a cloth, and let sit 45 minutes. Remove from sink and punch down. Place dough in lightly greased bread pan, and put in oven set at lowest possible setting, for further rising. When loaf has risen fully, set oven at 350° and bake 40 minutes, or until done. Cool on rack.

This delicious bread will become a favorite for family and friends. You might consider having a baker in your town bake you a large batch of 25 to 100 loaves at one time. He'll appreciate the business, and will do an excellent baking and slicing job for you. Divide the bread among friends or freeze it all away for yourself. (It will keep frozen indefinitely.) Once you've gotten the groundwork done with a local baker, you can get all the bread you need with a simple phone call. He may even deliver for you. (By the way, the bread is best when made from wheat ground into flour the same day it is baked into bread. Your baker can help you with that process, too.)

PITA BREAD
Level 3
(1 K-cup = ½ pita)

When pita bread is put into the oven, it is in the form of a round slab about the size of a slice of bread. This pita round bakes only a few minutes, and in that time it begins to puff up. Its surfaces puff apart, leaving a handy space inside the pita that is ideal for stuffing, sandwich-style. When a pita round has finished cooking, a slice may be made at its edge, gaining entry to the pocket inside. Or it may be snipped in two, making two stuffable pockets. Stuff it with leftover meat loaf, beans and cheese, taco stuffing, or any other sandwich makings desired.

1 envelope active dry yeast   3 cups whole wheat flour
3 cups white flour

In a large bowl or pot, sprinkle yeast on 2 cups plus 2 tablespoons of lukewarm (105°) water. Let stand 10 minutes. Add whole wheat flour and stir in well. Add white flour, stir, then work with hands into a ball. On very lightly floured board (use 3 tablespoons flour for flouring board), knead dough about 5 minutes, or until smooth and elastic. Shape into a ball. Place in a flour-dusted bowl, cover with damp paper towel or cloth towel, and put in a warm place to rise. If necessary, remoisten towel. When dough has doubled, shape and stretch into a long roll. Cut in 16 pieces. Gently toss pieces in hands to round them into ball shapes, and place them on a clean, dry, flour-dusted cloth. Cover with dry paper towels, and let rise 30 minutes. Roll each ball into a flat circle no thicker than ¼ inch. Turn dough over, place on dry, flour-dusted towels, and let rise 30 minutes. Place each round, top side down, directly on oven rack or wire rack. Dough should not be sticky or wrinkled on rack. If necessary, flip dough several times on floured board to dry before placing on oven rack. Bake at 475° until pitas puff (usually less than 5 minutes). Immediately transfer to broiler and brown tops. Cool on cake racks, then store in plastic bag till needed. Makes 16 pitas.

WATER BAGELS
Level 3
(1 K-cup = 1 bagel)

1 envelope active dry yeast
1 cup lukewarm (105°)
  potato water (water in
  which peeled potatoes
  have been cooked)

2½ to 3 cups flour
1 egg white

Soften yeast 10 minutes in potato water. Stir in 1 cup flour, blending until very smooth, then stir in remaining flour until dough can be handled. Turn out onto floured board and knead 10 minutes or until smooth and elastic, adding flour while kneading to make a firm dough. Place dough in floured, nonstick casserole dish. Cover and let rise until double in bulk. Turn dough out, punch down, and knead until smooth. On floured surface, roll out dough and cut into 16 pieces. With hands, roll each piece into a 5-inch-long log. Shape log into donut, moistening ends to join. Let rise 15 minutes on well-floured board. Drop bagels into boiling water, a few at a time. Let each bagel boil for 1 minute, then turn and boil 3 minutes on other side. Remove bagels with slotted spoon and place on cookie sheet. Brush with a mixture of slightly beaten egg white and 1 tablespoon water. Bake at 425° until crusts are light brown and crisp (about 25 minutes). Great with **Cream Cheese.** Makes 16 bagels.

DESSERTS

FRESH FRUIT DESSERT
Level 2
(1 K-cup = ½ cup)

½ watermelon (cut lengthwise)
1 cantaloupe
½ pound seedless grapes
4 bananas, sliced

4 peaches, sliced
½ fresh pineapple, cut in
  chunks
6 sprigs fresh mint

Remove inside of watermelon with a melon scoop. Sawtooth the edge of the melon. Cut and clean the cantaloupe and use a melon scoop to get as much of the fruit as possible. Toss all fruit (except bananas) gently in watermelon shell and chill. When ready to serve, add bananas and toss lightly. Garnish with mint sprigs. Serves 6 to 10.

ICE CREAM PIE
Level 2
(1 K-cup = 2" × 3" slice)

¾ cup apple juice
¾ cup nonfat dry milk
2 bananas, sliced

2 cups frozen blueberries
2 cups frozen strawberries
2½ cups Grape-Nuts

Combine apple juice and dry milk, and beat with electric mixer until whipped (works faster if bowl, beater, and ingredients are icy cold). Pour half of whipped mixture into blender, and blend with fruit, a little at a time, until thick and of an even consistency. Add to remaining half of whipped mixture and mix well. Add 1½ cups of the Grape-Nuts and mix well again. Moisten remaining Grape-Nuts and flatten into a layer on the bottom of 2 pie pans. Pour pie mixture into pans and freeze (about 2 hours). Makes 2 pies.

BUTTERMILK CHIFFON CHEESECAKE
Level 3
(1 K-cup = 3" × 4" slice)

FILLING:

4½ cups dry-curd cottage cheese *or* **Sour Cream**
1 cup **Buttermilk**
One 6-ounce can of frozen apple juice concentrate
2 tablespoons unflavored gelatin

One 8-ounce can of unsweetened crushed pineapple
1 teaspoon vanilla
3 egg whites, beaten to stiffness

CRUST:

Grape-Nuts

TOPPING (optional):

One 20-ounce package of frozen strawberries

1 tablespoon cornstarch

Make filling: Loosely crumble cottage cheese into blender. Add buttermilk and blend until very smooth. Thoroughly dissolve the can of frozen apple juice in 2 cans water. If contents of blender appear too dry, add a few tablespoons of the apple juice to blender and blend. Combine gelatin and pineapple in large bowl and mix well. Heat 1 cup of the apple juice to boiling, pour over gelatin and pineapple mixture, and stir to dissolve gelatin. Set aside to cool. Beat egg whites to stiffness. Add vanilla and the contents of the blender to the cooled pineapple-gelatin mixture, then fold in egg whites.

Make crust: Dampen enough Grape-Nuts with apple juice to cover bottom and sides of two 9-inch pie pans.

Make Topping (optional): Place strawberries in saucepan. Blend cornstarch with 2 tablespoons apple juice, combine with remaining apple juice (should be about ¾ to ⅞ cup), and add to saucepan. Bring to boil, reduce heat to medium-low, and cook until thickened.

Assemble cheesecakes: Pour filling into pie pan, spooning some over middle to make nice rounded form. Spread on topping and refrigerate until firm (about 1 hour). Makes 2 cheesecakes.

ORANGE SHERBET
Level 3
(1 K-cup = ½ cup)

One 6-ounce can of frozen   ⅔ cup nonfat dry milk
   orange juice concentrate   3 drops vanilla
1½ cups skim milk

Combine all ingredients in blender and blend until well mixed. Place in freezer until firm. Serve topped with fresh fruit and Grape-Nuts for crunch. Makes 1½ pints sherbet.

BLUEBERRY SAUCE
Level 2
(1 K-cup = ½ cup)

1 cup clear apple juice   1 cup frozen whole
2 teaspoons cornstarch   blueberries

Mix apple juice and cornstarch in small saucepan until lump-free. Add berries and cook, stirring constantly, over moderate heat until sauce clears and thickens, mashing berries while stirring. Serve hot over pancakes. Makes 1½ cups.

Optional: When sauce is ready to serve, stir in an additional ½ cup of frozen berries. Use this cooled sauce over pancakes or reheat slightly, stirring gently to avoid crushing berries.

STRAWBERRY SAUCE
Level 2
(1 K-cup = ½ cup)

1 cup apple juice   1 cup mashed strawberries
2 teaspoons cornstarch   ½ cup sliced strawberries

In a small saucepan, combine apple juice and cornstarch until lump-free. Add mashed berries, and cook over low-to-moderate heat, stirring constantly, until thickened, red, and bubbly. Add sliced berries just before serving over pancakes. Makes 2 cups.

APPLE BAKE
Level 3
(1 K-cup = 2″ × 3″ slice)

4 cups fresh apple slices	1 teaspoon cornstarch
2 tablespoons raisins	½ teaspoon cinnamon
1 tablespoon lemon juice	(½ cup rolled oats)
¼ cup apple juice	(½ cup Grape-Nuts)

Toss apple slices with raisins, lemon juice, and 1 tablespoon water. Set aside. Combine apple juice, cornstarch, and cinnamon with ½ cup water and cook, stirring constantly, until clear and slightly thickened. Spread rolled oats evenly over bottom of baking dish. Combine thickened sauce and apples and pour over oats. Top with Grape-Nuts and bake at 300° until apples are very tender (about 40 minutes). The oats and Grape-Nuts give the dish a delightful crust-and-crumb-pie effect, but may be omitted. When omitted, this dish may be served by itself, or it may be served over pancakes. Serves 8.

LUCINDA'S GRAIN DESSERT
Level 4
(1 K-cup = 3″ × 3″ slice)

One 23-ounce package uncooked mixed-grain cereal
(e.g., 7-Grain or 4-Grain)
One 15-ounce can juice-packed pineapple slices
2 cups apple juice *or* pineapple juice
1 cup water

Mix cereal, apple juice, and water together in an 11″ × 14″ glass baking dish. Place pineapple slices on top and bake 20 minutes at 350°. Serve in bowls, with skim milk as topping for those desiring it. Serves 12.

Answers to Problems in Chapter 5 (pages 77–78)

Problem 1: Most of the ingredients in Zowie Cereal are unacceptable. The unacceptable ingredients are: sugar, salt, coconut oil, and artificial flavor. To date, the preservative BHT has not been shown to be harmful to animals or people—you have to make up your own mind on this ingredient. The vitamins and mineral ingredients in this cereal are a danger sign for two reasons. First, they signal that the processing of the food has probably depleted the food of important nutrients, that must now be added back. Second, they signal the possibility of vitamin overdosage. On a diet of longevity foods, which is naturally rich in vitamins and minerals, added nutrients can create unwanted excess.

Problem 2: All the ingredients in this muffin mix are unacceptable except the nonfat dry milk. The bleached white flour is unacceptable because the complex nature of the carbohydrate of the natural whole flour is partially lost in the bleaching and refining of the flour. The other unacceptable ingredients are sugar, shortening, egg yolk, salt, and artificial colors and flavors.

Problem 3: Buttermilk Biscuit Mix is too high in fat: 100 times the grams of fat is 800 (100 $\times$ 8 = 800). And 800 is more than the 240 total calories in a serving.

Problem 4: French rolls are *not* too high in fat: 100 times the grams of fat is 100 (100 $\times$ 1 = 100), which is exactly equal to the 100 total calories in a serving.

SOURCE NOTES

Source Notes

Introduction

Page
1   "In the labs . . . percent overweight." A. Sclafani and D. Springer, "Dietary Obesity in Rats," *Physiology and Behavior* 17 (1976): 461–71.

2   "Sims and his . . . day indefinitely." E. A. H. Sims et al., "Endocrine and Metabolic Effects of Experimental Obesity in Man," *Recent Progress in Hormone Research* 29 (1973): 457–96.

2   "The fact that . . . years ago." H. P. Himsworth, "Physiological Activation of Insulin." *Clinical Science* 1 (1933): 1–38.

3   "The satiety center's . . . the blood . . . " A. F. Debons and I. Krimsky, "Insulin Requirements for Satiety Center Activity," in *Obesity Symposium,* Samuel Burland et al., eds. (New York: Churchill-Livingstone, 1974), pp. 146–59.

3   ". . . and the rate . . . the body." B. K. Anand, "Neurological Mechanisms Regulating Appetite," ibid., pp. 116–45.

3   "In 1950 Neal . . . been destroyed." N. E. Miller, C. J. Bailey and J. A. F. Stevenson, "Decreased 'Hunger' but Increased Food Intake Resulting from Hypothalamic Lesions," *Science* 112 (1950): 256–59.

4   "Schacter and his . . . normal weight." S. Schacter, L. N. Friedman, and J. Handler, "Who Eats with Chopsticks?" in *Obese Humans and Animals,* S. Schacter and J. Rodin, eds. (Potomac, Maryland: Lawrence Erlbaum Associates, 1974), pp. 61–64.

4   "In another study . . . normal weight." S. A. Hashim and T. B. Van Itallie, "Studies with Normal and Obese Subjects with a Monitored Food Dispensing Device," *Annals of the New York Academy of Science* 131 (1965): 654–61.

4   "The Bantus of . . . from sugar." A. R. P. Walker, B. F. Walker and B. D. Richardson, "Glucose and Fat Tolerances in Bantu Children," *The Lancet* (4 July 1970), p. 51.

4 "Connor and his . . . blood pressure." W. E. Connor et al., "The Plasma Lipids, Lipoproteins, and Diet of the Tarahumara Indians of Mexico," *American Journal of Clinical Nutrition* 31 (1978): 1131–42.

5 "In 1962 Srole . . . were overweight." L. Srole et al., *Mental Health in the Metropolis: The Midtown Manhattan Study*, rev. ed. in 2 vols. (New York: Harper and Row, 1975).

5 "A study of . . . traditionally (unacculturated)." A. J. Stunkard, J. L. Garb and J. R. Garb, "Social Factors and Obesity in Navajo Indian School Children," in *Recent Advances in Obesity Research: I*, A. Howard, ed. (Westport, Connecticut: Technomic Publishing Co., 1974), pp. 37–39.

5 "Oscanova, who is . . . general population." K. Oscanova, "Trends of Dietary Intake and Prevalence of Obesity in Czechoslovakia," *Recent Advances in Obesity Research: I*, A Howard, ed. (Westport, Connecticut: Technomic Publishing Co., 1974), pp. 42–44.

6 "In Nigeria, fats . . . those ages." B. K. Adadevoh, "Obesity in the African," in *Obesity Symposium*, Samuel Burland et al., eds. (New York: Churchill-Livingstone, 1974), pp. 60–73.

6 "Kuzuya and his . . . tolerance tests." T. Kuzuya, M. Irie and Y. Niki, "Glucose Intolerance among Japanese Professional Sumo-Wrestlers," in *Diabetes Mellitus in Asia*, Baba, Goto and Fukui, eds. (Amsterdam: Excerpta Medica, 1976), pp. 137–44.

Chapter 1: Read This Chapter First

Page
10 " '. . . most obese patients . . . it promptly.' " Cornell Conferences on Therapy, "Management of Obesity," *New York State Journal of Medicine* 58 (1958): 79–87.

Chapter 3: Roving

Page
28 "In 1954 Jean . . . pounds overweight.)" J. Mayer et al., "Exercise, Food Intake and Body Weight in Normal Rats and Genetically Obese Adult Mice," *American Journal of Physiology* 77: 544–48.

30   "Dr. Mayer showed . . . sedentary workers." J. Mayer, P. Roy and K. P. Mitra, "Relation between Caloric Intake, Body Weight, and Physical Work," *American Journal of Clinical Nutrition* 4 (1956): 169–75.

32   "In 1970 Bjorntorp . . . and dramatic." P. Bjorntorp, "The Effects of Exercise on Human Obesity," in *Obesity Symposium,* Samuel Burland et al., eds. (New York: Churchill-Livingstone, 1974), pp. 171–91.

33   "Dr. U. D. Register . . . on the BMR." U. D. Register, "Keeping Your Calorie Bank in Balance," *Life and Health* 2 (1974): 46–47.

34   "As early as . . . exercise session." D. E. Gray and A. deVries, "After-Effects of Exercise on Metabolic Rate," *The Research Quarterly* 34 (1963): 314–19. Published by the American Association for Health, Physical Education and Recreation in affiliation with the National Education Association, Washington, D.C.

35   "Dr. Charles W. Frank . . . less active." C. W. Frank et al., "Physical Inactivity as a Lethal Factor in Myocardial Infarction in Men," *Circulation* 34 (1966): 1022–33.

35   "Ralph Paffenbarger of . . . heart attack." R. S. Paffenbarger, "Physical Activity and Fatal Heart Attack: Protection or Selection?" in *Exercise in Cardiovascular Health and Disease,* Ezra A. Amsterdam et al., eds. (New York: Yorke Medical Books, 1977), pp. 35–52.

36   "For example, John . . . these people." J. S. Hanson et al., "Long Term Physical Training and Cardiovascular Dynamics in Middle-Aged Men," *Circulation* 38 (1968): 783–99.

36   "Jack Wilmore . . . by 1 percent." J. H. Wilmore, "Individualized Exercise Prescription," in *Exercise in Cardiovascular Health and Disease,* Ezra A. Amsterdam et al., eds. (New York: Yorke Medical Books, 1977), pp. 267–73.

38   "Dr. Melvin Williams . . . exercise format.' " M. H. Williams, *Nutritional Aspects of Human Physical and Athletic Performance* (Springfield, Illinois: C. C. Thomas Publishers, 1976), p. 269.

38   "Duddleston and Bennion . . . mental attitude.' " A. K. Duddleston and M. Bennion, "Effect of Diet and/or Exercise on Obese College Women," *Journal of the American Dietetic Association* 56 (1970): 126–29.

38   "Czechoslovakia has started . . . less depression." J. Sonka, "Effects of Diet or Diet and Exercise in Weight Reducing Regimens in Czechoslovakia," in *Nutrition, Physical Fitness, and Health,* Parizkova and Rogozkin, eds. (Baltimore, Maryland: University Park Press, 1978), pp. 239–47.

39   "Dr. Robert Brown . . . significant level.' " R. Brown, quoted in
      Runner's World Magazine (January 1978), p. 41.
39   Mensen Ernst of . . . in all. Norris McWhirter, *Guinness Book of
      World Records* (New York: Sterling Publishing Co., 1979), p.
      659.

Chapter 4: Jogging and Running

Page
41   "According to Dr. John . . . run regularly." J. D. Cantwell,
      "When Friends and Patients Ask about Running," *Journal of the
      American Medical Association* 240 (1978): 1409–10.
41   "Dr. George Sheehan . . . the universe.' " George Sheehan, "The
      Basics of Jogging," *Runner's World Magazine* (August 1977),
      pp. 34–36.
42   "According to an . . . to strangers." In "Tarahumarans, a Tribe
      that Fascinates Cardiology and Psychiatry," *Journal of the
      American Medical Association* 208 (1969): 1617 and 1624.
42   "As W. E. . . . . the Tarahumarans." W. E. Connor et al., "The
      Plasma Lipids, Lipoproteins, and Diet of the Tarahumara Indians
      of Mexico," *American Journal of Clinical Nutrition* 31 (1978):
      1131–42.
43   "Begin running by . . . 4 weeks." George Sheehan, "The Basics
      of Jogging," *Runner's World Magazine* (August 1977), pp.
      34–36.
50   "And as Dr. . . . . made available.' " J. H. Wilmore, "Indi-
      vidualized Exercise Prescription," in *Exercise in Cardiovascular
      Health and Disease*, Ezra A. Amsterdam et al., eds. (New York:
      Yorke Medical Books, 1977), pp. 267–73.

Chapter 7: Two Weeks to Go: Data Gathering and Practice

Page
96   "R. B. Stuart has . . . nearest competitor." R. B. Stuart, *Slim
      Chance in a Fat World* (Champaign, Illinois: Research Press,
      1972).

Chapter 8: One Week to Go: Adaptation

Page

109   "Vivienne Aries of . . . practically nil." V. Aries, "Bacteria and the Etiology of Cancer of the Large Bowel," *Gut* 10 (1969): 334–35.

109   "USDA researchers Kelsay, . . . 38 hours." J. L. Kelsay, K. M. Behall and E. S. Prather, "Effects of Fiber from Fruit and Vegetables on Metabolic Responses of Human Beings," *American Journal of Clinical Nutrition* 31 (1978): 1149–53.

109   "In his study . . . 9.5 hours." A. R. P. Walker, "Effect of High Crude Fiber Intake on Transit Time and the Absorption of Nutrients in South African Schoolchildren," *American Journal of Clinical Nutrition* 28 (1975): 1161–69.

109   "Inferred from Walker's . . . following morning." D. P. Burkitt, A. R. P. Walker and N. S. Painter, "Effect of Dietary Transit Fiber on Stools and Transit Times, and Its Role in the Causation of Disease," *The Lancet* (30 December 1972), pp. 1408–12.

110   "Hernias are thought . . . Western foods." T. P. Almy, "Diverticulosis," in *Textbook of Medicine,* Paul B. Beeson and Walsh McDermott, eds. 13th ed. (Philadelphia: W. B. Saunders Company, 1971), pp. 1257 and 1258.

GENERAL INDEX

General Index

RECIPE INDEX

Recipe Index

NOTES

NOTES

NOTES